THE ANTI-INFLAMMATORY PSORIASIS DIET COOKBOOK

The All-in-One Guide to Total Healing from Symptoms, Treatment, and Prevention of Similar Diseases

Audrey McAllister, MD

Copyright © 2024 Audrey McAllister, MD

must be accompanied by appropriate attribution and citation to the original source.

Requests for permission to use or reproduce any part of this publication should be addressed to the publisher in writing. The publisher reserves the right to grant or deny permission at their discretion, taking into consideration factors such as the intended use, nature of the excerpt, and potential impact on the original work.

Unauthorized reproduction or distribution of copyrighted material is a violation of intellectual property rights and may result in legal consequences. Individuals or entities found to be in breach of copyright law may be subject to legal action, including but not limited to injunctions, damages, and legal fees.

Table of Contents

INTRODUCTION TO PSORIASIS

Psoriasis stands as a formidable challenge for those who grapple with its manifestations. It emerges as an autoimmune condition, unleashing skin inflammation that can significantly disrupt one's quality of life. Esteemed dermatologists worldwide frequently encounter individuals affected by this prevalent skin disorder, with statistics indicating its prevalence in roughly 2% of the population in the United States alone.

While genetic predisposition plays a significant role in the onset and severity of psoriasis, environmental factors such as infections or trauma also exert considerable influence. Stress, although not directly responsible for triggering psoriasis, can undoubtedly exacerbate its symptoms, exacerbating the discomfort and distress experienced by those afflicted.

Characterized by the emergence of red, raised, and scaly patches across the skin, psoriasis knows no bounds concerning age or gender. Its presence can provoke incessant itching and discomfort, rendering affected individuals vulnerable to a myriad of emotional and psychological challenges. While it bears no contagious nature, the visible nature of psoriatic lesions can induce feelings of embarrassment and significantly undermine one's self-confidence, particularly in social settings.

Typically, psoriasis presents itself in a symmetrical pattern across the scalp, lower back, elbows, and knees, though its reach can extend to various other areas of the skin. Nail involvement, regions behind the ears, or along the hairline are not exempt from its impact, adding to the multifaceted nature of its symptoms. Thickened, discolored patches of skin adorned with scales characterize the clinical presentation of psoriasis, with these plaques serving as poignant reminders of its chronicity.

The burden of psoriasis extends beyond the physical realm, encroaching upon the emotional and mental well-being of those affected. Its chronic nature, coupled with the absence of a definitive cure, underscores the importance of effective management strategies. Psoriasis can induce pain, disrupt sleep patterns, and impede cognitive function, perpetuating a cycle of discomfort and distress.

Triggers for psoriasis flare-ups are diverse, ranging from infections to physical trauma and certain medications, particularly in individuals with a genetic predisposition to the condition. However, amidst the challenges posed by psoriasis, there exists a glimmer of hope in the form of available treatments and lifestyle adjustments. Through a tailored approach encompassing both medical interventions and holistic coping strategies, individuals can embark on a journey towards a more fulfilling life despite the presence of psoriasis. By embracing a proactive stance and harnessing the support of healthcare professionals, one can navigate the complexities of psoriasis with resilience and determination, forging a path towards enhanced well-being and self-empowerment.

daily activities and negatively impact mental well-being.

In essence, psoriasis represents more than just a skin condition; it is a complex interplay of immune dysfunction, genetic predisposition, and environmental factors. Understanding the underlying mechanisms of psoriasis sheds light on the challenges faced by those living with the condition and underscores the importance of comprehensive management approaches aimed at addressing both the physical and emotional aspects of the disease.

What Is Psoriasis?

Psoriasis emerges as a multifaceted autoimmune condition, intricately woven with genetic predispositions, that orchestrates an accelerated pace of skin cell proliferation. This accelerated growth cycle gives rise to the formation of scaly, crimson-hued skin lesions that often ignite sensations of discomfort, ranging from a mild itch to a burning sensation. Typically making its debut on the skin canvas between the tender ages of 15 and 25, psoriasis stands as a pervasive challenge, affecting the lives of over 8 million individuals in the United States alone and surpassing a staggering toll of 125 million worldwide.

Within the taxonomy of psoriasis, one encounters a diverse spectrum of manifestations, each bearing its own unique characteristics and clinical presentations. Among these variants are plaque, guttate, inverse, pustular, and erythrodermic psoriasis, each offering its own distinct narrative within the broader tale of this dermatological disorder. Plaque psoriasis, the unrivaled protagonist in this narrative, presents itself with raised lesions adorned in a white mantle of dead skin cells, reminiscent of an artistic tableau crafted upon the skin's canvas. Conversely, alternate types may evoke images of crimson, lustrous lesions or eruptive pustules, each contributing its own chapter to the unfolding saga of psoriasis.

However, amidst this taxonomy, one encounters a sinister protagonist, known as erythrodermic psoriasis, whose presence casts a shadow over the narrative with its unparalleled severity. This formidable form can blanket the majority of the body in a relentless siege, inflicting excruciating pain upon its bearer and orchestrating a dramatic symphony of skin peeling, leaving a trail of physical and emotional wreckage in its wake. In the face of such a formidable adversary, those grappling with psoriasis find themselves embroiled in a daily struggle, navigating not only the physical manifestations but also the profound psychological toll exacted by this relentless condition.

The difference between psoriasis and eczema

Experiencing the persistent annoyance of an itch that seems to have a mind of its own is undoubtedly one of the most exasperating sensations. It's like an uninvited guest that just won't take the hint to leave. Often, this itchiness is not just a fleeting inconvenience but a symptom of underlying skin conditions that can disrupt daily life and wreak havoc on one's comfort.

Among the common culprits of such relentless itching are psoriasis and eczema, two skin disorders that share the common denominator of causing discomfort through itching, dryness, and the development of rashes that stubbornly resist fading away. These conditions can turn even a simple scratch into a trigger for redness and inflammation, leaving those affected caught in a cycle of discomfort and frustration.

Despite their similar outward appearances, psoriasis and eczema possess distinct characteristics that are crucial for both sufferers and medical professionals to recognize. Understanding these nuances can significantly aid in accurate diagnosis and, subsequently, effective treatment plans tailored to address the specific needs of each condition.

Psoriasis, for instance, is often characterized by the rapid buildup of skin cells, resulting in thick, silvery scales and red patches. On the other hand, eczema typically manifests as inflamed, itchy patches of skin that may ooze or become crusty over time. By discerning these subtle yet significant disparities, individuals afflicted by these conditions can better navigate their journey toward relief and improved skin health.

Moreover, delving into the underlying causes of psoriasis and eczema unveils a complex interplay of genetic predisposition, environmental factors, and immune system dysfunction. While genetic factors predispose some individuals to these conditions, triggers such as stress, allergens, and climate can exacerbate symptoms, exacerbating the itch-scratch cycle and intensifying discomfort.

Navigating the labyrinth of treatment options for psoriasis and eczema requires a tailored approach that addresses both symptom management and underlying causes. From topical creams and ointments to phototherapy and systemic medications, there exists a spectrum of interventions aimed at alleviating itching, reducing inflammation, and promoting skin healing.

Furthermore, embracing holistic strategies such as stress management techniques, dietary modifications, and skincare rituals can complement conventional treatments, fostering a comprehensive approach to skin health and overall well-being. By integrating these multifaceted approaches, individuals grappling with psoriasis and eczema can embark on a path toward long-term relief and a restored sense of comfort in their own skin.

In essence, while nothing quite compares to the frustration of dealing with a relentless itch, understanding the nuances of skin conditions like psoriasis and eczema empowers individuals to take proactive steps toward managing symptoms and reclaiming control over their skin health. By fostering awareness, embracing tailored treatments, and prioritizing self-care, the itch-scratch cycle can be broken, paving the way for a brighter, itch-free future.

The various kinds of psoriasis

Psoriasis, a chronic autoimmune condition, manifests in various forms, each presenting unique challenges and symptoms. One of the most prevalent types is plaque psoriasis, affecting a significant majority of individuals with this condition. Plaque psoriasis, scientifically termed Psoriasis Vulgaris, derives its name not from any vulgarity but rather from its widespread occurrence. This type typically manifests as dry, itchy patches of raised skin, often covered in scales, which can vary in size and severity. These patches commonly appear on the elbows, knees, lower back, and scalp, exhibiting different colors depending on the individual's skin tone.

In contrast, inverse psoriasis tends to affect skin folds, such as those found in the groin, buttocks, and breasts. Unlike plaque psoriasis, it presents as smooth, inflamed patches of skin without scales, exacerbated by friction and sweating. Furthermore, fungal infections can exacerbate this type of psoriasis, adding another layer of complexity to its management.

Guttate psoriasis, often triggered by streptococcal infections like sore throat, manifests as small, red, drop-shaped scaly spots on the skin. It predominantly affects children and young adults, posing challenges not only for the individual but also for parents grappling with the sudden onset of this condition in their child. While treatable, its appearance can be alarming and may raise concerns about long-term implications.

Pustular psoriasis, on the other hand, presents with small, pus-filled bumps atop plaques, representing a rarer manifestation of the condition. This form can lead to clearly defined blistering, occurring in patches on the palms or soles, adding to the diversity of symptoms experienced by individuals with psoriasis.

Erythrodermic psoriasis, the least common but most severe form, can cover more than 90% of the body, resulting in widespread skin discoloration and shedding. This condition, whether acute or chronic, manifests as a peeling rash that can cause intense itching or burning, significantly impacting quality of life.

Sebopsoriasis, a hybrid of psoriasis and seborrheic dermatitis, primarily affects the face and scalp, characterized by bumps and plaques with a greasy, yellow scale. Additionally, nail psoriasis can lead to changes in nail appearance, including pitting, abnormal growth, discoloration, and detachment from the nail bed, which can significantly impact manual dexterity and self-esteem.

The diverse manifestations of psoriasis underscore the complexity of this condition and the importance of personalized treatment approaches tailored to address individual symptoms and concerns. Moreover, ongoing research and medical advancements hold promise for improved management strategies and enhanced quality of life for those living with psoriasis.

SECTION 2: SIGNS AND SYMPTOMS OF PSORIASIS

The signs and symptoms of psoriasis encompass a spectrum of manifestations that vary from individual to individual, reflecting the complex nature of this dermatological condition. One of the hallmark indicators is the emergence of a patchy rash, whose appearance can differ significantly, ranging from dandruff-like scaling spots to extensive eruptions that may engulf substantial portions of the body. These rashes may exhibit a diverse array of colors, appearing purple with a gray scale on darker skin tones, or pink or red with a silver scale on lighter skin tones, thus adding to the intricacy of its presentation.

Moreover, individuals with psoriasis may experience spots of minor scaling, particularly observable in children, alongside skin that is characterized by dryness, cracking, and even occasional bleeding. The discomfort associated with psoriasis often extends beyond physical manifestations, with patients frequently reporting sensations of itching, burning, or pain, further complicating their quality of life. Additionally, the cyclic nature of the rash, wherein it may intermittently appear and disappear over the course of weeks or months, adds a layer of unpredictability and frustration for those affected.

Furthermore, the classification of psoriasis into distinct types—plaque, guttate, inverse, pustular, and erythrodermic—underscores the heterogeneity of this condition and highlights the varying symptoms associated with each subtype. For instance, plaque psoriasis, the most prevalent form, typically manifests as itchy, red, thick, scaly patches predominantly observed on the knees, elbows, lower back, or scalp. In contrast, guttate psoriasis is characterized by the development of small red spots on the trunk or limbs, often triggered by bacterial or viral infections, thereby illustrating the multifaceted nature of its etiology.

Furthermore, the clinical presentation of psoriasis can be particularly severe and potentially life-threatening in the case of erythrodermic psoriasis, wherein the patient's skin assumes a bright red hue, accompanied by increased heart rate and difficulty in maintaining normal body temperature. Prompt medical intervention becomes imperative in such instances to mitigate the associated risks.

Importantly, it is essential to dispel misconceptions surrounding the contagious nature of psoriasis, as it cannot be transmitted through interpersonal contact. While the exact cause of psoriasis remains elusive, a combination of genetic predisposition and environmental triggers is thought to underlie its pathogenesis. These triggers encompass a broad spectrum, ranging from infections, skin injuries, and stress to lifestyle factors such as smoking, excessive alcohol consumption, vitamin D deficiency, and certain medications, thereby highlighting the multifactorial nature of this condition.

Furthermore, the intricate interplay between psoriasis and psoriatic arthritis, affecting nearly 30% of individuals with psoriasis, further underscores the systemic nature of this disease. Psoriatic arthritis is typified by joint pain, stiffness, and swelling, often punctuated by periods of exacerbated symptoms known as flares, thereby accentuating the profound impact of psoriasis on both dermatological and musculoskeletal health.

In essence, the diverse array of signs and symptoms associated with psoriasis underscores the multifaceted nature of this condition, necessitating a comprehensive understanding of its clinical manifestations and underlying mechanisms to facilitate effective management and improve patient outcomes.

Things That Can Make Psoriasis Worse

For individuals who possess a genetic predisposition to psoriasis, the onset of symptoms may remain latent for an extended period before environmental factors trigger the manifestation of the disease. This delay in symptom presentation can often lead to a false sense of security, as individuals may be unaware of their susceptibility until a triggering event occurs. Psoriasis, a chronic autoimmune condition characterized by the rapid proliferation of skin cells, can be incited by various environmental triggers, each capable of sparking an immune response and exacerbating the condition.

Among the common triggers for psoriasis are microbial infections such as streptococcal throat infections and skin infections. These infections can instigate an inflammatory response within the body, thereby prompting the onset or worsening of psoriatic symptoms. Additionally, weather conditions, particularly cold and dry climates, have been identified as significant triggers for psoriasis flare-ups. The lack of moisture in the air and harsh environmental elements can cause skin dryness and irritation, exacerbating the symptoms of psoriasis.

Furthermore, physical trauma to the skin, whether it be a minor cut, scrape, insect bite, or severe sunburn, can serve as a catalyst for psoriatic lesions to develop or worsen. The disruption of the skin barrier can trigger an immune response, leading to inflammation and the rapid turnover of skin cells characteristic of psoriasis.

Behavioral factors such as smoking and exposure to secondhand smoke have also been implicated in the exacerbation of psoriatic symptoms. The harmful chemicals present in tobacco smoke can disrupt immune function and contribute to systemic inflammation, thereby worsening psoriasis severity.

Moreover, excessive alcohol consumption has been linked to the exacerbation of psoriasis, likely due to its detrimental effects on immune function and inflammatory pathways. Certain medications, including lithium, blood pressure medications, and antimalarial drugs, have also been identified as potential triggers for psoriatic flare-ups. These medications can disrupt immune regulation and contribute to the development or exacerbation of psoriasis symptoms.

Additionally, the abrupt discontinuation of oral or injected corticosteroids, commonly used to manage psoriatic symptoms, can paradoxically lead to a rebound effect, causing a sudden worsening of psoriasis symptoms known as steroid withdrawal flare.

What puts you at risk for psoriasis?

Psoriasis, a chronic autoimmune condition characterized by red, scaly patches on the skin, doesn't discriminate – it can affect individuals across all age groups and walks of life. Surprisingly, approximately one-third of all psoriasis cases manifest during childhood, emphasizing the importance of understanding its risk factors and triggers early on.

One significant influencer in the development of psoriasis is one's family history. The genetic component of psoriasis is undeniable, as it tends to run in families. Having a parent with psoriasis already increases the likelihood of developing the condition, but if both parents are affected, the risk escalates even further. This underscores the interplay between genetics and environmental factors in determining an individual's susceptibility to psoriasis.

Moreover, lifestyle choices play a crucial role in exacerbating the risk and severity of psoriasis. Smoking, in particular, has been identified as a significant contributor. Tobacco use not only heightens the likelihood of developing psoriasis but can also exacerbate existing symptoms, leading to more frequent flare-ups and potentially worsening the overall prognosis. Understanding the detrimental effects of smoking on psoriasis underscores the importance of adopting healthier habits to manage the condition effectively.

In essence, while psoriasis may seem like a random occurrence, delving deeper reveals the intricate web of genetic predisposition and environmental influences at play. By acknowledging these factors and making informed lifestyle choices, individuals can take proactive steps towards mitigating their risk of developing psoriasis or managing its symptoms more effectively if already diagnosed.

SECTION 3: WHAT CAUSES PSORIASIS?

Psoriasis, a chronic skin condition, is instigated by an immune system that's kicked into overdrive, sparking inflammation across the skin's surface. Picture it like a bustling construction site, where certain areas of your skin are working overtime, producing new cells at a pace that's far speedier than the norm. This frenetic activity manifests as dry, scaly patches, creating a visibly uncomfortable appearance.

Moreover, the affected regions experience a surge in blood flow, resulting in a telltale redness and swelling, as if your skin is staging a protest against this immune system uprising. And it doesn't stop there. Sometimes, this inflammatory process can extend its reach into your joints, triggering pain, swelling, and stiffness—a condition known as psoriatic arthritis, adding a layer of complexity to the already burdensome symptoms.

Now, when you're living with psoriasis, your immune system, like a vigilant guardian, is supposed to sniff out and eliminate foreign invaders like bacteria, all in the noble pursuit of keeping you healthy and illness-free. However, in a curious twist of fate, it can sometimes misidentify perfectly healthy cells as hostile intruders.

Thus begins a relentless onslaught of inflammation and swelling, culminating in the formation of those telltale skin plaques. Normally, your skin cells undergo a patient 30-day journey from creation to shedding. But with psoriasis, this timeline is dramatically expedited, thanks to your immune system's overzealousness, pushing out new cells every three to four days instead. Consequently, you're left with a constant cycle of scales and frequent skin shedding atop these inflamed patches, making for a visually and physically discomforting experience.

Furthermore, psoriasis isn't just a skin-deep issue; it often carries a hereditary component. It's like a genetic hand-me-down, where biological parents might unwittingly pass down this condition to their offspring, adding an extra layer of complexity and potential concern to family health histories.

What triggers psoriasis flare-ups?

A psoriasis flare-up, often referred to as an outbreak, occurs due to exposure to triggers, which can range from irritants to allergens. These triggers vary from person to person, making the experience of psoriasis flare-ups highly individualized. Common factors known to provoke psoriasis flare-ups include:

1. Emotional stress: Heightened emotional tension can act as a catalyst for psoriasis flare-ups, exacerbating the condition in susceptible individuals. Stress management techniques may help mitigate its impact.

2. Infections: Certain infections, such as streptococcal infections, have been identified as potential triggers for psoriasis flare-ups. Maintaining good hygiene practices and promptly addressing infections can aid in managing the condition.

3. Skin trauma: Any form of skin injury, whether it be a cut, scrape, or surgical procedure, has the potential to trigger a psoriasis flare-up in affected individuals. Careful handling of the skin and prompt treatment of injuries are essential preventative measures.

4. Medications: Some medications, including lithium and beta-blockers, have been linked to exacerbating psoriasis symptoms in certain individuals. It is crucial for patients to discuss potential side effects with their healthcare providers and explore alternative treatment options if necessary.

5. Weather changes: Fluctuations in weather conditions, particularly shifts in body temperature, can influence the severity of psoriasis symptoms. Extreme temperatures, humidity levels, and seasonal changes may trigger flare-ups in susceptible individuals, necessitating adjustments in skincare routines and environmental modifications.

Understanding and identifying these triggers can empower individuals living with psoriasis to take proactive measures in managing their condition and minimizing the frequency and severity of flare-ups. Through a combination of lifestyle modifications, stress management techniques, and medical interventions, individuals can strive to achieve better control over their psoriasis symptoms and improve their overall quality of life.

Challenges Arising from Psoriasis

If you happen to be grappling with psoriasis, it's essential to recognize that this condition often comes hand in hand with a myriad of other potential health challenges. Among these are the distinctive symptoms of psoriatic arthritis, where individuals may experience joint discomfort, stiffness, and swelling, which can significantly impact mobility and quality of life.

Additionally, as the skin undergoes the cyclical process of flare-ups and healing, it may exhibit temporary alterations in coloration, such as post-inflammatory hypopigmentation or hyperpigmentation, particularly in areas where plaques have resolved.

Beyond the realm of dermatological concerns, psoriasis can cast its shadow over ocular health, potentially leading to conditions like conjunctivitis, blepharitis, and uveitis, underscoring the systemic nature of this disorder.

The ramifications extend further into the realm of systemic health, as individuals with psoriasis may find themselves at a heightened risk for comorbidities such as obesity, type 2 diabetes mellitus, and hypertension, all of which can exert a substantial toll on overall well-being.

Moreover, the inflammatory nature of psoriasis can reverberate throughout the body, manifesting in cardiovascular complications and predisposing individuals to a spectrum of autoimmune maladies. These may include celiac disease, sclerosis, and Crohn's disease, each presenting its own set of challenges and management considerations.

Not to be overlooked are the profound effects that psoriasis can have on mental health. It's not uncommon for individuals grappling with this condition to experience a diminished sense of self-esteem and an increased susceptibility to depression, underscoring the importance of holistic care that addresses both the physical and psychological dimensions of well-being.

In essence, navigating life with psoriasis entails not just managing its visible manifestations but also remaining vigilant to its potential systemic implications and prioritizing comprehensive care that addresses the interconnected facets of health.

Here's some friendly advice to help you keep psoriasis at bay!

Ensuring your skin remains adequately moisturized is pivotal in managing psoriasis, as symptoms tend to exacerbate when the skin becomes dry. Utilizing moisturizing lotions, with petroleum jelly often considered the most effective, forms a cornerstone of this regimen. By diligently applying these lotions, you create a protective barrier, preventing excessive dryness that can trigger flare-ups.

Moreover, adopting a gentle approach toward your skin and scalp is imperative. Avoid the temptation to pick at dried scales, as doing so may further irritate the condition. Even seemingly innocuous actions like trimming your nails can pose risks; any cuts incurred during this process can potentially worsen your symptoms. Consistent bathing with prescribed products aids in maintaining control over the condition, serving as another essential aspect of your skincare routine.

Weather extremes represent another factor to consider. Excessive exposure to sunlight, cold temperatures, or dry weather conditions can all instigate flare-ups. Therefore, taking precautions to shield your skin from such extremes becomes crucial in managing psoriasis effectively.

Furthermore, managing your weight is paramount, as obesity significantly contributes to skin flare-ups. By maintaining a healthy weight through balanced nutrition and regular exercise, you can mitigate this risk factor and potentially alleviate symptoms.

Addressing lifestyle habits is also key. Tobacco use in any form has been shown to aggravate psoriasis, necessitating a proactive approach to cessation. Whether it involves quitting smoking or chewing tobacco, taking steps to eliminate this habit can greatly improve prevention efforts.

Additionally, consulting with your doctor is essential in understanding the specific triggers that may cause flare-ups for you. It could be certain medications or dietary factors, and identifying and avoiding these triggers at all costs is imperative for effective management.

In summary, a comprehensive approach to managing psoriasis encompasses various strategies, from skincare practices and lifestyle modifications to seeking professional guidance. By prioritizing moisturization, gentle skincare routines, weather awareness, weight management, tobacco cessation, and trigger identification, you can significantly reduce the frequency and severity of flare-ups, thereby improving your overall quality of life.

SECTION 4: DEALING WITH PSORIASIS: HOW TO TACKLE IT

If you're coping with psoriasis, you might find yourself navigating a plethora of therapeutic options designed to manage the condition's symptoms and mitigate its impact on your skin and overall well-being. Psoriasis therapies span a spectrum of approaches, from topical treatments like creams and ointments to light therapy (phototherapy), and even oral or injectable medications.

The choice of therapy depends on various factors, including the severity of your psoriasis and how responsive it has been to previous treatments and self-care methods. Often, finding the right therapy involves a process of trial and error, where you may need to explore multiple medications or combinations of therapies before settling on what works best for you.

Even after finding an effective therapy, psoriasis can have a tendency to recur, necessitating ongoing management and vigilance.

Let's delve into the world of topical treatments, which are frequently the first line of defense against mild to moderate psoriasis. Corticosteroids, for instance, are commonly recommended for their anti-inflammatory properties. They come in various forms, including creams, ointments, lotions, and sprays, and can be tailored to suit different areas and severities of psoriasis. However, prolonged use of corticosteroids can lead to skin thinning and reduced effectiveness over time.

Vitamin D analogs, such as calcipotriene and calcitriol, offer another avenue for topical treatment by slowing down skin cell growth. These medications can be used alone or in combination with corticosteroids, providing an alternative or adjunct therapy for managing psoriasis symptoms.

Retinoids, like tazarotene, function by suppressing skin cell proliferation and are available in gel or cream formulations. While effective, they can cause skin discomfort and increased sensitivity to light, making them unsuitable for certain individuals, particularly those who are pregnant or planning to become pregnant.

Inhibitors of calcineurin, such as tacrolimus and pimecrolimus, offer a targeted approach to reducing scale accumulation and soothing skin inflammation, particularly in sensitive areas like the face and around the eyes where other treatments may be less tolerable or safe.

Salicylic acid, derived from plants, can help minimize scaling in psoriasis when used in shampoos or scalp treatments, facilitating the absorption of other topical medications.

Coal tar, anthralin, and phototherapy represent additional modalities for managing psoriasis, each with its own unique benefits and considerations. Coal tar, for instance, reduces scaling, irritation, and inflammation, but its strong odor and potential for skin irritation make it less appealing to some individuals. Anthralin, meanwhile, suppresses skin cell proliferation and can be effective in eliminating scales, albeit with the caveat of skin irritation and staining.

Phototherapy, whether through exposure to sunlight or artificial light sources like UVB or UVA, offers a versatile and widely used approach to treating psoriasis, either alone or in combination with other therapies. However, it requires careful monitoring to minimize the risk of adverse effects like inflammation and increased sun sensitivity.

For individuals with moderate to severe psoriasis unresponsive to topical treatments or phototherapy, oral or injectable medications may be recommended. These systemic therapies encompass a range of options, including steroids, retinoids, biologics, and immunosuppressants, each with its own efficacy profile and potential side effects. Biologics, for instance, target specific components of the immune system to disrupt the disease cycle and alleviate symptoms, but they can also increase the risk of infections and require careful monitoring.

In addition to conventional therapies, alternative approaches like special diets, vitamins, acupuncture, and herbal products have garnered interest among individuals seeking complementary or adjunctive treatments for psoriasis. While not supported by robust evidence, these alternative therapies are generally considered safe and may offer relief for some individuals, particularly those with mild to moderate symptoms.

When considering treatment options for psoriasis, it's essential to consult with your healthcare provider to develop a personalized plan that aligns with your needs and preferences. Together, you can explore the full spectrum of therapies available and weigh the potential benefits and drawbacks of each approach to optimize your management strategy.

Beyond medical interventions, self-care measures play a crucial role in managing psoriasis and promoting skin health. Simple practices like bathing with gentle cleansers, moisturizing regularly, and using humidifiers to combat dry air can help alleviate symptoms and maintain skin hydration. Covering affected areas with moisturizers overnight can also enhance the efficacy of topical treatments and reduce scaling.

In conclusion, managing psoriasis requires a multifaceted approach that encompasses medical therapies, lifestyle modifications, and self-care practices tailored to individual needs. By working closely with healthcare providers and adopting a holistic approach to treatment, individuals with psoriasis can effectively manage their condition and improve their quality of life.

Exploring Ways to Treat Your Condition

Eczema and psoriasis, two chronic dermatological conditions, demand sustained attention and management over the long term. The approach to treatment is multifaceted, contingent upon the severity of symptoms and the extent as well as the localization of the affected areas on the skin. Various therapeutic modalities exist, ranging from topical anti-inflammatories and moisturizing emollients to phototherapy and biologic or systemic medications, all aimed at modulating the body's inflammatory and immune responses to mitigate the symptoms.

Beyond merely exploring treatment options with your healthcare provider, it is paramount to be mindful of potential triggers or exacerbating factors that may precipitate or aggravate your symptoms. Factors such as humidity, allergens, and specific cleansers, soaps, and detergents have the potential to exacerbate eczema. Similarly, psoriasis flare-ups may be prompted not only by skin trauma but also by stress or infections.

Initiating the journey towards resolution of your skin afflictions begins with seeking professional medical evaluation and diagnosis. Although both eczema and psoriasis are characterized by their chronic nature, identifying and implementing the appropriate treatment regimen can significantly alleviate symptoms and diminish the frequency and severity of flare-ups. By proactively engaging with healthcare providers and adopting lifestyle modifications tailored to your individual needs, you can effectively manage these conditions and optimize your skin health and overall well-being in the long term.

Which areas of the body can psoriasis affect?

Psoriasis, a chronic autoimmune condition, manifests as a rash that can appear virtually anywhere on your body, presenting a diverse array of affected areas. Typically, it is commonly found on easily observable regions such as the knees and elbows, where plaques—thickened, red patches of skin—are frequently observed. Yet, its reach extends beyond these visible areas, potentially emerging in unexpected places like your face and even the inside of your mouth, where it can cause discomfort and disruption.

The scalp serves as another common site for psoriatic involvement, often leading to flaking and itchiness, which can be particularly bothersome. Additionally, the condition may extend its influence to the delicate regions of your finger and toe nails, resulting in pitting, discoloration, and even separation from the nail bed, posing both aesthetic and functional challenges.

Moreover, psoriasis can intrude upon intimate areas, affecting the genitals and potentially causing significant distress and sensitivity. It's not just limited to the extremities and visible surfaces; the lower back, palms, and soles of the feet are also susceptible to its effects, complicating everyday activities and comfort.

While psoriasis typically affects only small areas of the skin initially, in severe cases, these isolated patches can amalgamate, covering extensive portions of your body with thick, scaly plaques. This not only intensifies the physical discomfort but also amplifies the emotional toll, as the condition becomes more conspicuous and intrusive, affecting various aspects of daily life and self-image.

Can you catch psoriasis from someone else?

No, psoriasis is not something you can catch from another person. It doesn't spread through contact with someone else's skin rash. It's essential to understand that psoriasis isn't contagious; it doesn't transfer from one person to another like a common cold or flu. Rather, psoriasis is a chronic autoimmune condition where the immune system mistakenly attacks healthy skin cells, causing them to reproduce at an accelerated rate.

Individuals with psoriasis often face misconceptions and stigma due to misunderstandings about the condition. They don't need avoidance; they need empathy and support. Avoiding contact with someone with psoriasis won't prevent the condition from spreading because it simply doesn't spread that way. However, ostracizing or keeping a distance from them can have detrimental effects on their mental and emotional well-being.

Psoriasis patients require understanding and compassion more than anything else. By educating ourselves and others about the realities of psoriasis, we can create a more inclusive and supportive environment for those living with this chronic condition. Instead of fear or avoidance, let's offer kindness, acceptance, and assistance to individuals battling psoriasis.

SECTION 5: WHAT'S THE DEAL WITH PSORIATIC ARTHRITIS?

Psoriatic arthritis, a condition that can impact as many as 30% of individuals diagnosed with psoriasis, presents a complex interplay of symptoms and challenges. While a definitive cure remains elusive, acquiring a comprehensive understanding of this disorder and being equipped with knowledge regarding its potential manifestations can significantly alleviate the burden of pain, stress, and fatigue associated with it.

At its core, psoriatic arthritis constitutes an inflammatory form of arthritis, characterized by joint pain, swelling, and stiffness, particularly pronounced during the morning hours. Its etiology is closely intertwined with psoriasis or a familial predisposition towards the skin condition. Both psoriasis and psoriatic arthritis belong to the category of chronic autoimmune disorders, wherein certain cells within the body turn against its own tissues and cells, triggering a cascade of inflammatory responses.

The spectrum of psoriatic arthritis spans a wide range of severity, manifesting in various clinical presentations. Oligoarticular psoriatic arthritis describes a condition affecting four or fewer joints within the body, while polyarticular psoriatic arthritis extends its reach to involve four or more joints. Additionally, there exists a less common subtype known as spondylitis, primarily affecting the spine, hips, and shoulders, leading to further complications in mobility and functionality.

Who might end up grappling with Psoriatic Arthritis?

Psoriasis, a chronic autoimmune condition, impacts a significant portion of the global population, estimated to afflict around 2-3% of people worldwide, which translates to approximately 7 million individuals within the United States alone. This condition manifests in various forms, with one notable complication being the development of psoriatic arthritis, affecting up to 30% of those diagnosed with psoriasis.

Psoriatic arthritis tends to predominantly affect adults within the age range of 35 to 55, although it is important to note that it can emerge at any stage of life.

Both men and women are susceptible to this condition, indicating its impartiality towards gender.

Interestingly, psoriatic arthritis can arise independently of a prior diagnosis of psoriasis, with some individuals experiencing its onset solely based on a familial predisposition to psoriasis. Moreover, while less common, instances have been documented where psoriatic arthritis precedes the visible symptoms of psoriasis, challenging conventional assumptions about the sequential presentation of these conditions.

Moreover, there exists a notable intergenerational pattern in the transmission of psoriasis and its associated arthritis, with children born to parents affected by psoriasis being three times more likely to develop psoriasis themselves. Furthermore, these children are also at an increased risk of developing psoriatic arthritis, underscoring the complex genetic interplay underlying the inheritance of these conditions.

In the case of juvenile onset psoriatic arthritis, it is noteworthy that the most prevalent age range for its emergence is typically between 9 and 11 years old, emphasizing the importance of early detection and intervention in pediatric cases. This underscores the imperative for heightened vigilance and proactive management strategies, particularly in younger populations, to mitigate the long-term impact of psoriatic arthritis on physical health and overall quality of life.

What are the telltale signs and symptoms of psoriatic arthritis?

Psoriatic arthritis, a condition intertwined with both skin inflammation and joint discomfort, manifests itself in a myriad of ways across its afflicted patients. For some, the onset of symptoms is a gradual, almost imperceptible progression, while for others, the emergence can be abrupt and startling, disrupting their lives in unforeseen ways.

The spectrum of psoriatic arthritis symptoms is as diverse as the individuals it affects. From mild manifestations, subtly affecting a single joint, to severe instances where multiple joints are engulfed in distress, the variability is vast. Remarkably, not every patient experiences the complete array of symptoms, further complicating diagnosis and management.

When it comes to joint symptoms, aching, tenderness, and swelling become unwelcome companions for many. These sensations frequently target areas such as the hands, feet, wrists, ankles, and knees, encroaching upon the ease of everyday movement. Joint stiffness, particularly pronounced in the morning or after prolonged periods of rest, imposes its unwelcome presence, often serving as a persistent reminder of the condition's grip. Additionally, the affected joints' range of motion becomes notably restricted, adding another layer of impediment to one's mobility.

The discomfort doesn't stop there; lower back pain or stiffness can also rear its head, compounding the already burdensome symptoms. Furthermore, tenderness, pain, or swelling at the juncture where tendons and ligaments connect to bone, known as enthesitis, can exacerbate the overall distress, particularly evident in areas like the Achilles tendon in the heel. In more severe cases, the swelling of an entire digit, resembling a sausage, clinically termed dactylitis, becomes a visible marker of the condition's impact.

On the skin front, psoriatic arthritis often leaves its mark in the form of scaly silver or gray patches, commonly found on the scalp, elbows, knees, and lower spine. Papules, small raised spots often accompanied by scaling, may grace the arms, legs, and torso, further adding to the dermatological manifestation. Notably, nail pitting, characterized by tiny depressions, or detachment and lifting of fingernails or toenails, serve as additional clues to the underlying condition.

Beyond the realms of joints and skin, psoriatic arthritis can infiltrate other bodily systems, presenting with ocular inflammation, fatigue, and anemia. These additional symptoms, though not always immediately associated with the condition, underscore its systemic nature, affecting various aspects of a patient's well-being.

In essence, psoriatic arthritis is a multifaceted condition, showcasing a diverse array of symptoms that can significantly impact an individual's quality of life. Its nuanced presentation underscores the importance of personalized treatment approaches tailored to address the unique needs of each patient.

What leads to Psoriatic Arthritis?

Psoriatic arthritis remains a condition shrouded in mystery, its origins elusive within the intricate dance of genetic predispositions and environmental triggers. Scientists grapple with the intricate web spun between hereditary factors and external influences, all while considering the nuanced interplay of immune system dysregulation, potential infections, the burden of weight, and the impact of physical trauma on susceptibility to this condition. Unlike a contagious malady, psoriasis and its arthritic counterpart are not spread through contact but emerge from within the body's own systems.

In a recent breakthrough study, researchers uncovered a compelling link between psoriatic arthritis and elevated levels of tumor necrosis factor (TNF) found within the affected joints and skin regions of afflicted individuals. These heightened levels of TNF present a formidable challenge to the immune system, overwhelming its capacity to quell the inflammation associated with the manifestations of psoriatic arthritis. This discovery sheds light on a potential pathway through which the disease manifests, offering new avenues for therapeutic intervention and a deeper understanding of its pathogenesis.

SECTION 6: HOW IS PSORIATIC ARTHRITIS DIAGNOSED?

Psoriatic arthritis remains a condition shrouded in mystery, its origins elusive within the intricate dance of genetic predispositions and environmental triggers. Scientists grapple with the intricate web spun between hereditary factors and external influences, all while considering the nuanced interplay of immune system dysregulation, potential infections, the burden of weight, and the impact of physical trauma on susceptibility to this condition. Unlike a contagious malady, psoriasis and its arthritic counterpart are not spread through contact but emerge from within the body's own systems.

In a recent breakthrough study, researchers uncovered a compelling link between psoriatic arthritis and elevated levels of tumor necrosis factor (TNF) found within the affected joints and skin regions of afflicted individuals. These heightened levels of TNF present a formidable challenge to the immune system, overwhelming its capacity to quell the inflammation associated with the manifestations of psoriatic arthritis. This discovery sheds light on a potential pathway through which the disease manifests, offering new avenues for therapeutic intervention and a deeper understanding of its pathogenesis.

Dealing with Psoriatic Arthritis

Diagnosing psoriatic arthritis isn't a straightforward process that hinges on a single test; rather, it's a comprehensive evaluation conducted by healthcare practitioners such as medical doctors, osteopathic physicians, nurse practitioners, and physician assistants. This diagnostic journey typically involves a thorough review of the patient's medical history, a meticulous physical examination, an array of blood tests, and occasionally, X-rays of the affected joints. While magnetic resonance imaging (MRI) is rarely needed except in extreme cases, a combination of these diagnostic tools helps paint a clearer picture of the condition.

Laboratory tests play a crucial role in aiding diagnosis and monitoring disease activity. Among these are blood tests such as rheumatoid factor and anti-cyclic citrullinated peptide (anti-CCP), which assist in diagnosing rheumatoid arthritis. Additionally, the HLA-B27 blood test may be recommended, especially if there's a familial history of psoriasis or psoriatic arthritis. Markers of inflammation like erythrocyte sedimentation rate (ESR) and C-reactive protein (CRP) levels provide valuable insights into disease activity.

In the early stages of the illness, X-rays might not reveal conclusive evidence of psoriatic arthritis. However, as the disease progresses, X-rays can uncover characteristic alterations typically associated with psoriatic arthritis. For instance, the "pencil-in-cup" deformity, where the end of the bone erodes into a sharp point, is one such hallmark. These radiographic findings indicate more severe inflammatory changes within the joints, potentially necessitating more aggressive therapeutic interventions.

If you're experiencing both psoriasis and arthritis symptoms, confirming a diagnosis of psoriatic arthritis becomes somewhat more straightforward for your healthcare provider. However, it's essential to note that symptoms of psoriatic arthritis may manifest independently of psoriasis in up to 15% of individuals. Given the variability of symptoms from one patient to another, it's crucial to maintain open communication with your healthcare provider, especially if symptoms worsen or new ones emerge. Consulting with a healthcare professional ensures timely intervention and appropriate management strategies tailored to your specific needs.

What treatment choices are available for psoriatic arthritis?

The primary objective of therapeutic interventions for psoriatic arthritis is twofold: to effectively manage the condition and to alleviate associated symptoms. This entails a multifaceted approach, often involving a combination of pharmaceutical and non-pharmaceutical modalities tailored to each individual's needs.

When it comes to pharmaceutical interventions, several classes of medications are commonly employed. Disease-modifying antirheumatic drugs (DMARDs), such as Methotrexate, Sulfasalazine, and Cyclosporine, represent a cornerstone in the pharmacological management of psoriatic arthritis. However, in cases where nonsteroidal anti-inflammatory drugs (NSAIDs) or traditional DMARDs fail to adequately control the disease, biologic agents emerge as a viable treatment option. Since their introduction in 2005, biologics have demonstrated remarkable efficacy in not only slowing down disease progression but also in preventing joint deterioration.

Before initiating any pharmaceutical regimen, thorough laboratory testing and discussions about safety considerations with a healthcare provider are imperative. Proper management of psoriatic arthritis and associated psoriasis is crucial not only for symptom control but also for mitigating systemic risks, notably cardiovascular complications.

Complementing pharmaceutical interventions, various non-pharmacological strategies can play a significant role in managing joint discomfort and improving overall quality of life.

Regular exercise, tailored to individual capabilities and preferences, can help alleviate joint stiffness and discomfort associated with psoriatic arthritis. Physical or occupational therapy-guided range-of-motion and strengthening exercises, when combined with low-impact aerobics, can be particularly beneficial. It's essential to consult with a healthcare professional before starting any new exercise regimen to ensure its appropriateness and safety.

Incorporating heat and cold therapy into the daily routine can also provide relief. Alternating between moist heat, such as warm towels or baths, and cold therapy, like ice packs, can help reduce pain, swelling, and stiffness in affected joints.

Adopting joint protection and energy conservation techniques in daily activities can minimize stress on joints and reduce fatigue. Practicing good body mechanics and maintaining proper posture are vital for preserving joint function and conserving energy. Individuals with psoriatic arthritis are encouraged to vary positions frequently during work, home, and leisure activities to prevent joint strain.

In some cases, healthcare providers may recommend splinting to alleviate inflammation or address concerns regarding joint alignment or stability. Splints should be periodically removed to facilitate joint movement, accompanied by gentle range-of-motion exercises.

While surgery is rarely necessary for most individuals with psoriatic arthritis, severe joint damage or injury may warrant joint replacement surgery. The goal of surgical intervention is to restore function, alleviate discomfort, improve mobility, or enhance the physical appearance of the affected area. However, it's important to explore surgical options only when conservative measures have been exhausted and the benefits outweigh the risks.

What treatment option suits me best?

The course of treatment prescribed to manage your condition hinges upon the severity of your symptoms at the time of diagnosis, aiming to effectively control the disease and achieve a state of remission while mitigating potential complications. As the condition progresses, there might be a necessity to adjust medications to sustain effective management and stave off disease progression and systemic effects. Early indicators of a more severe disease manifestation include an early onset, involvement of multiple joints, and spinal complications, underscoring the importance of attentive monitoring.

In the therapeutic journey of psoriatic arthritis, the health of your skin assumes paramount importance. Thus, a comprehensive approach often involves consultations with two distinct healthcare providers, typically a rheumatologist and a dermatologist. Early detection and intervention play pivotal roles in alleviating pain and inflammation while forestalling further joint deterioration and associated damage. Left untreated, psoriatic arthritis can escalate into a disabling condition, perpetuating chronic pain, compromising quality of life, and heightening the risk of cardiovascular complications.

Vigilance in observing changes in symptoms and responsiveness to medication is crucial. Promptly informing your healthcare provider of any shifts in your condition or ineffectiveness of your current medication regimen ensures timely adjustments and optimized management strategies. This collaborative effort between patient and healthcare team is essential in navigating the complexities of psoriatic arthritis and fostering improved outcomes and well-being.

SECTION 7:   DIETARY TIPS EVERYONE SHOULD BE AWARE OF

Living with psoriasis can present significant challenges, particularly when the manifestations of the condition are visible to others or affect a substantial portion of your body. The discomfort and embarrassment that often accompany this chronic skin condition can be overwhelming. Additionally, the ongoing nature of psoriasis, coupled with the hurdles associated with its treatment, can further compound the burden it imposes on individuals.

Navigating life with psoriasis requires a multifaceted approach aimed at fostering a sense of control and empowerment. One essential aspect of this journey is educating oneself about psoriasis. By delving into comprehensive knowledge about the condition and exploring available treatment options, individuals can better understand their own circumstances and make informed decisions about managing their health. It's crucial to identify potential triggers that may exacerbate flare-ups and take proactive measures to mitigate their impact.

Furthermore, fostering a support network is invaluable in coping with the emotional and psychological toll of psoriasis. Sharing experiences and connecting with others who are facing similar challenges can provide solace and encouragement. Whether through local support groups or online communities, finding solidarity with fellow individuals navigating psoriasis can offer invaluable support and validation.

In addition to seeking support from peers, adhering to the guidance of healthcare professionals is paramount. Following medical advice regarding treatment regimens and lifestyle adjustments can significantly impact the management of psoriasis symptoms. It's essential to communicate openly with healthcare providers, asking questions and seeking clarification when needed to ensure optimal care.

For many individuals, managing the visible effects of psoriasis on their appearance can be a source of insecurity and self-consciousness. Utilizing cover-ups such as clothing or cosmetic concealers can offer a sense of control on days when self-esteem is particularly challenged. However, it's essential to exercise caution with these products to avoid exacerbating skin irritation, especially on open wounds or inflamed areas.

Moreover, acknowledging the potential role of stress in triggering psoriasis flare-ups underscores the importance of prioritizing emotional well-being. While the exact relationship between stress and psoriasis remains complex and merits further research, adopting stress-reducing practices can contribute to symptom management. Engaging in activities that promote relaxation and mindfulness, such as meditation, yoga, or spending quality time with loved ones, can help alleviate stress and cultivate a sense of balance amidst the challenges of living with psoriasis.

Can Changing Your Diet Help Treat Psoriasis?

Certainly, as indicated by dermatologist Anthony Fernandez, MD, PhD, especially if one is dealing with obesity or is categorized as overweight, there is compelling evidence suggesting that reducing weight through a hypocaloric (low-calorie) dietary regimen can significantly ameliorate the overall severity of psoriasis. Taking into account not only the quantity but also the quality of food consumed is paramount when modifying one's dietary habits. It's crucial to recognize that the impact of dietary choices extends beyond mere caloric intake; the specific nutritional composition of foods plays a vital role in influencing the physiological processes underlying psoriasis manifestation. Hence, adopting a balanced and nutrient-rich dietary approach can potentially yield favorable outcomes in managing psoriasis symptoms and promoting overall skin health.

What are some foods that people with psoriasis should steer clear of?

Encountering compilations delineating specific trigger foods to steer clear of if you happen to be grappling with psoriasis is quite common. Nevertheless, as underscored by Dr. Fernandez, blindly adhering to such directives isn't always imperative. "By and large, we don't counsel individuals with psoriasis to categorically eschew particular dietary items." In numerous instances, this leniency stems from the absence of concrete scientific substantiation linking specific foods to psoriasis flare-ups. Dr. Fernandez, for instance, accentuates the lack of evidence suggesting eggs might incite a flare-up.

However, there might be occasions when you subjectively perceive certain foods to exert an influence on your psoriasis. "We frequently encounter individuals who report, 'I sense my psoriasis flares up if I consume this specific type of food,'" Dr. Fernandez adds. In such scenarios, it's prudent to pay heightened attention to how your body reacts after consuming said meal, either by monitoring its impact or opting to abstain from it entirely, and assessing any discernible differences over time.

"We are always open to experimenting with minor, innocuous adjustments like that," Dr. Fernandez elucidates. "Each person is unique and may have an individualized trigger for their condition. If any concerns are raised, we take them seriously." That being said, Dr. Fernandez underscores that there exists a spectrum of foods that could potentially exacerbate psoriasis.

Meals laden with high levels of fat or sugar warrant caution. While body fat is indispensable for overall health, its surplus can incite inflammation, which is detrimental for psoriasis. Dr. Fernandez advises steering clear of calorically dense meals that heighten the likelihood of accruing body fat—essentially, fried fast food and sugary confections.

Alcohol consumption also merits moderation. "It's established that individuals who indulge in alcohol are more predisposed to developing psoriasis," elucidates Dr. Fernandez. "However, abstaining from alcohol may not always yield significant long-term improvement in illness." Instead, adhering to your physician's recommendations regarding alcohol consumption without overindulgence is prudent.

Do psoriasis vitamins provide relief? You might have come across assertions suggesting that incorporating substances with anti-inflammatory properties, such as turmeric, could ameliorate psoriasis symptoms. However, scientific validation may not consistently corroborate such claims. "If we're unsure whether excessive intake of this supplement could yield adverse effects, we typically advise, 'Go ahead and try it,'" he adds. "However, there is currently insufficient empirical evidence to support the notion that any specific nutrients can alleviate psoriasis."

Can changing what you eat help with managing psoriasis?

Managing psoriasis involves more than just adhering to a specific diet regimen, as emphasized by Dr. Fernandez. In navigating treatment options, it becomes evident that there is no universally optimal diet tailored specifically for every patient battling psoriasis. The complexity lies in the multifaceted nature of this condition, where dietary adjustments alone might not suffice to alleviate symptoms entirely, necessitating complementary medical interventions.

Dr. Fernandez underscores the nuanced approach required, highlighting that while dietary modifications can play a role in managing psoriasis, they are rarely the standalone solution. It's crucial to recognize that for many individuals, achieving significant improvement solely through dietary changes is unlikely, warranting the inclusion of other therapeutic modalities.

However, amidst this acknowledgment, certain dietary patterns exhibit more pronounced efficacy in mitigating psoriasis symptoms than others. Understanding these nuances empowers patients and healthcare providers to tailor treatment strategies holistically, encompassing dietary adjustments alongside pharmacological interventions and lifestyle modifications. Through this comprehensive approach, individuals grappling with psoriasis can optimize their management plan to enhance overall well-being and symptom control.

CHAPTER 8: PSORIASIS MEALS: MORNING, NOON, EVENING, GREENS, BROTH, AND HOTPOT IDEAS

DELICIOUS MORNING MEAL IDEAS

Low-Carb Bacon Spinach Egg Cups

Things You Need

cooking spray

4 slices thick-cut bacon, diced

½ (12 ounce) package frozen chopped spinach, thawed and drained

4 mushrooms, chopped

¼ green bell pepper, chopped

2 slices onion, chopped

1 pinch salt and ground black pepper to taste

6 eggs

1 tablespoon heavy whipping cream

1 ¼ cups shredded Colby-Jack cheese, divided

½ teaspoon salt

¼ teaspoon ground black pepper

1 pinch onion powder

1 pinch garlic powder

Instructions

Preheat oven to 350 degrees F (175 degrees C). Spray 12 muffin cups with cooking spray.

Cook and stir bacon in a skillet over medium-high heat until crisp, about 10 minutes. Transfer bacon to a bowl, reserving bacon grease in the skillet.

Combine spinach, mushrooms, green bell pepper, onion, salt, and ground black pepper to taste in the skillet with bacon grease; cook and stir until softened, about 5 minutes. Transfer vegetable mixture to a bowl and place in the freezer to cool, about 5 minutes.

Whisk eggs and cream together in a bowl; stir in 1 cup Colby-Jack cheese, 1/2 teaspoon salt, 1/4 teaspoon ground black pepper, onion powder, and garlic powder. Add cooled vegetables and bacon to egg mixture and mix gently.

Scoop 1/4 cup egg mixture into each muffin cup; top each with remaining Colby-Jack cheese.

Bake in the preheated oven until egg cups are set, about 20 minutes.

Cook's Notes: Substitute any cooked meat or any cooked veggie. Make sure if you're low carbin' it, that they are low-carb ingredients though. Cheddar cheese can be used in place of Colby-Jack, if desired. I use silicone muffin cups, but the greased muffin tin is fine.

Eggs and Greens Breakfast Dish

Things You Need

1 tablespoon olive oil

2 cups stemmed and chopped rainbow chard

1 cup fresh spinach

½ cup arugula

2 cloves garlic, minced

4 eggs, beaten

½ cup shredded Cheddar cheese

salt and ground black pepper to taste

Instructions

Heat oil in a skillet over medium-high heat. Saute chard, spinach, and arugula until tender, about 3 minutes. Add garlic; cook and stir until fragrant, about 2 minutes.

Mix eggs and cheese together in a bowl; pour into the chard mixture. Cover and cook until set, 5 to 7 minutes. Season with salt and pepper.

Cook's Note: You can substitute Cheddar cheese with any shredded cheese of your choice.

Breakfast Chickpea Spinach Muffins

Things You Need

2 tablespoons coconut oil

1 (10 ounce) package frozen spinach, thawed

2 eggs

1 (15 ounce) can chickpeas, rinsed and drained

½ cup nutritional yeast

¼ cup grated Parmesan cheese

1 teaspoon ground paprika

salt and ground black pepper to taste

Instructions

Preheat oven to 375 degrees F (190 degrees C). Grease a muffin tin with coconut oil.

Combine spinach and eggs in a food processor; pulse until blended. Add chickpeas; pulse until blended. Add nutritional yeast, Parmesan cheese, paprika, salt, and pepper; pulse until evenly incorporated.

Pour spinach mixture into the prepared muffin tin, filling each cup 2/3 full.

Bake in the preheated oven until a toothpick inserted into the center comes out clean, about 25 minutes.

Light and Fluffy Spinach Quiche

Things You Need

½ cup light mayonnaise

½ cup milk

4 large eggs, lightly beaten

1 (10 ounce) package frozen chopped spinach, thawed and sq ueezed dry

8 ounces shredded reduced-fat Cheddar cheese

¼ cup chopped onion

1 (9 inch) unbaked pie shell

Instructions

Preheat the oven to 400 degrees F (200 degrees C). Line a cookie sheet with foil.

Whisk together mayonnaise and milk in a large bowl until smooth. Whisk in eggs; set aside.

Layer spinach, cheese, and onion in the pie shell, making several layers of each. Place on the prepared cookie sheet. Slowly pour egg mixture into the pie shell, then cover q uiche with foil.

Bake in the preheated oven for 45 minutes. Uncover and continue baking until the top is golden brown and filling is set, 10 to 15 more minutes.

Mushroom Spinach Omelet

Things You Need

1 (8 ounce) carton liq uid egg substitute

1 tablespoon shredded Cheddar cheese

1 tablespoon shredded Parmesan cheese

¼ teaspoon salt

⅛ teaspoon ground black pepper

⅛ teaspoon garlic powder

⅛ teaspoon red pepper flakes

1 teaspoon olive oil

½ cup chopped fresh mushrooms

1 tablespoon chopped onion

½ cup chopped fresh spinach, or more to taste

Instructions

Whisk egg substitute, Cheddar cheese, Parmesan cheese, salt, black pepper, garlic powder, and red pepper flakes together in a bowl.

Heat olive oil in a nonstick skillet over medium heat; cook and stir mushrooms and onion until tender, 4 to 5 minutes. Add spinach; cook until spinach wilts, 3 to 4 minutes. Pour in egg mixture; swirl pan around to evenly distribute egg mixture. Cook until egg is fully cooked and set in the middle, 5 to 10 minutes. Cut into wedges.

Poached Eggs Caprese

Things You Need

1 tablespoon distilled white vinegar

2 teaspoons salt

4 eggs

2 English muffin, split

4 (1 ounce) slices mozzarella cheese

1 tomato, thickly sliced

4 teaspoons pesto

salt to taste

Instructions

Fill a large saucepan with 2 to 3 inches of water and bring to a boil over high heat. Reduce the heat to medium-low, pour in vinegar and 2 teaspoons of salt, and keep water at a gentle simmer.

While waiting for water to simmer, place a slice of mozzarella cheese and a thick slice of tomato onto each English muffin half, and toast in a toaster oven until cheese softens and English muffin has toasted, about 5 minutes.

Crack an egg into a small bowl. Holding the bowl just above water's surface, gently slip egg into simmering water. Repeat with remaining eggs. Poach eggs until whites are firm and yolks have thickened but are not hard, 2 1/2 to 3 minutes. Remove eggs from water with a slotted spoon and dab them on a kitchen towel to remove excess water.

To assemble, place a poached egg on top of each English muffin. Spoon a teaspoon of pesto sauce onto each egg and sprinkle with salt to taste.

Eggs and Greens Breakfast Dish

Things You Need

1 tablespoon olive oil

2 cups stemmed and chopped rainbow chard

1 cup fresh spinach

½ cup arugula

2 cloves garlic, minced

4 eggs, beaten

½ cup shredded Cheddar cheese

salt and ground black pepper to taste

Instructions

Heat oil in a skillet over medium-high heat. Saute chard, spinach, and arugula until tender, about 3 minutes. Add garlic; cook and stir until fragrant, about 2 minutes.

Mix eggs and cheese together in a bowl; pour into the chard mixture. Cover and cook until set, 5 to 7 minutes. Season with salt and pepper.

Cook's Note: You can substitute Cheddar cheese with any shredded cheese of your choice.

Caprese on Toast

Things You Need

14 slices sourdough bread

2 cloves garlic, peeled

1 pound fresh mozzarella cheese, sliced 1/4-inch thick

⅓ cup fresh basil leaves

3 large tomatoes, sliced 1/4-inch thick

3 tablespoons extra-virgin olive oil

salt and ground black pepper to taste

Instructions

Toast bread slices and rub one side of each slice with garlic. Place a slice of mozzarella cheese, 1 to 2 basil leaves, and a slice of tomato on each piece of toast. Drizzle with olive oil and season with salt and black pepper.

Mediterranean Breakfast Quinoa

Things You Need

¼ cup chopped raw almonds

1 teaspoon ground cinnamon

1 cup quinoa

2 cups milk

1 teaspoon sea salt

1 teaspoon vanilla extract

2 tablespoons honey

2 dried pitted dates, finely chopped

5 dried apricots, finely chopped

Instructions

Toast the almonds in a skillet over medium heat until just golden, 3 to 5 minutes; set aside.

Heat the cinnamon and q uinoa together in a saucepan over medium heat until warmed through. Add the milk and sea salt to the saucepan and stir; bring the mixture to a boil, reduce heat to low, place a cover on the saucepan, and allow to cook at a simmer for 15 minutes. Stir the vanilla, honey, dates, apricots, and about half the almonds into the q uinoa mixture. Top with the remaining almonds to serve.

Eggs Florentine

Things You Need

2 tablespoons butter

½ cup mushrooms, sliced

2 cloves garlic, minced

½ (10 ounce) package fresh spinach

6 large eggs, slightly beaten

salt and ground black pepper to taste

3 tablespoons cream cheese, cut into small pieces

Instructions

Melt butter in a large skillet over medium heat; cook and stir mushrooms and garlic until garlic is fragrant, about 1 minute. Add spinach to mushroom mixture and cook until spinach is wilted, 2 to 3 minutes.

Stir eggs into mushroom-spinach mixture; season with salt and pepper. Cook, without stirring, until eggs start to firm; flip. Sprinkle cream cheese over egg mixture and cook until cream cheese starts to soften, about 5 minutes.

Chef John's Shakshuka

Things You Need

2 tablespoons olive oil

1 large onion, diced

½ cup sliced fresh mushrooms

1 teaspoon salt, or more to taste

1 cup diced red bell pepper

1 jalapeno pepper, seeded and sliced

1 teaspoon cumin

½ teaspoon paprika

½ teaspoon ground turmeric

½ teaspoon freshly ground black pepper, plus more to taste

¼ teaspoon cayenne pepper

1 (28 ounce) can crushed San Marzano tomatoes, or other high-quality plum tomatoes

½ cup water, or more as needed

6 large eggs

2 tablespoons crumbled feta cheese

2 tablespoons chopped fresh parsley

Instructions

Heat olive oil in a large, heavy skillet over medium-high heat. Add onions and mushrooms. Sprinkle with salt. Cook and stir until mushrooms release all of their liq uid and start to brown, about 10 minutes. Stir in bell peppers and jalapeno pepper. Cook and stir until peppers begin to soften up, about 5 minutes. Season with cumin, paprika, turmeric, black pepper, and cayenne. Stir and cook to "wake up" the flavors, about 1 minute. Pour in crushed tomatoes and water. Adjust heat to medium and simmer uncovered until veggies are softened and sweet, stirring occasionally, 15 to 20 minutes. Add more water if sauce becomes too thick.

Make a depression in the sauce for each egg with a large spoon. Crack egg into a small ramekin and slide gently into each indentation; repeat with the rest of the eggs. Season with salt and pepper. Cover and cook until eggs are to your desired doneness.

Top with feta cheese and parsley.

Healthy Breakfast Sandwich

Things You Need

¾ cup liquid egg whites

2 whole-wheat English muffins, split

½ cup baby spinach leaves

2 slices fresh tomato

Instructions

Cook egg whites in a nonstick skillet over medium heat until opaque, about 4 minutes.

Toast English muffins. Divide cooked egg whites between 2 muffin bottoms. Top with spinach, 1 tomato slice, and muffin tops.

Spinach Feta Egg Wrap

Things You Need

1 large whole-wheat tortilla

1 ½ teaspoons coconut oil

1 cup chopped baby spinach leaves

1 oil-packed sun-dried tomato, chopped

2 eggs, beaten

⅓ cup feta cheese

1 tomato, diced

Instructions

Warm tortilla in a large skillet over medium heat.

Melt coconut oil in a separate skillet over medium-high heat. Sauté spinach and tomato in hot oil until spinach wilts, about 1 minute.

Add eggs and scramble until almost set, about 2 minutes. Sprinkle feta cheese over eggs and continue cooking until cheese melts, about 1 minute more.

Transfer scrambled egg mixture to warm tortilla in the large skillet; top with diced tomato. Roll tortilla and leave in skillet long enough for wrap to hold its shape, about 30 seconds.

Tips: Use butter instead of coconut oil if you want; you can also try tomato- and basil-flavored feta cheese.

Zucchini with Egg

Things You Need

1 ½ tablespoons olive oil

2 large zucchini, cut into large chunks

salt and ground black pepper to taste

2 large eggs

1 teaspoon water, or as desired

Instructions

Heat oil in a skillet over medium-high heat; saute zucchini until tender, about 10 minutes. Season zucchini with salt and black pepper.

Beat eggs with a fork in a bowl; add water and beat until evenly combined. Pour eggs over zucchini; cook and stir until eggs are scrambled and no longer runny, about 5 minutes. Season zucchini and eggs with salt and black pepper.

Paleo Baked Eggs in Avocado

Things You Need

2 small eggs

1 avocado, halved and pitted

2 teaspoons chopped fresh chives, or to taste

1 pinch dried parsley, or to taste

1 pinch sea salt and ground black pepper to taste

2 slices cooked bacon, crumbled

Instructions

Preheat the oven to 425 degrees F (220 degrees C).

Crack eggs into a bowl, being careful to keep the yolks intact.

Arrange avocado halves in a baking dish, resting them along the edge so avocado won't tip over. Gently spoon 1 egg yolk into the avocado hole. Continue spooning egg white into the hole until full. Repeat with remaining egg yolk, egg white, and avocado. Season each filled avocado with chives, parsley, sea salt, and pepper.

Gently place baking dish in the preheated oven and bake until eggs are cooked, about 15 minutes. Sprinkle bacon over avocado.

Scrumptious Breakfast Salad

Things You Need

5 eggs

1 head romaine lettuce, chopped

2 avocados, sliced

2 large tomatoes, sliced

1 pint fresh strawberries, sliced

4 clementines, peeled and segmented

1 Spanish onion, sliced into rounds

1 ripe mango, peeled and sliced

1 Pink Lady apple, diced

1 nectarine, sliced

1 cucumber, diced

¼ cup vinaigrette salad dressing, or to taste

Instructions

Place eggs in a saucepan and cover with water. Bring to a boil, remove from heat, and let eggs stand in hot water for 15 minutes.

Layer lettuce, avocados, tomatoes, strawberries, clementines, onion, mango, apple, nectarine, and cucumber in a large bowl or on individual serving plates. Drizzle vinaigrette on top.

Remove eggs from hot water; cool under cold running water. Peel and chop. Scatter eggs over the salad.

Cook's Notes: Omit whatever you choose. Another great option is to add thinly sliced steak or salmon. Beef or tuna carpaccio works well. Use a strawberry or apple cider vinaigrette if preferred.

IDEAS FOR A DELICIOUS LUNCH

Olive Oil Mashed Potatoes With Garlic

Things You Need

1½ pounds Yukon gold potatoes, q uartered

1 tablespoon sea salt, plus more to taste

¼ cup extra virgin olive oil

2 to 3 cloves of garlic, smashed, peeled, and kept whole

Black pepper, to taste

1-2 tablespoons flat-leaf parsley, chopped (optional)

Instructions

In a stockpot, add the potatoes and enough cold water to cover the potatoes by 1 inch. Add the salt and bring to a boil. Partially cover and simmer until very tender, about 15 minutes depending on their size. Reserve 1 cup of cooking water and drain.

Meanwhile, in a small pot on very low heat, warm the olive oil with the garlic cloves. Cook for 20 minutes, while keeping an eye on it to make sure the garlic does not burn (see Chef Tips). The garlic cloves should gradually turn a deep golden color. Remove and discard the garlic.

Return the drained potatoes to the stockpot, add the garlicky olive oil, a pinch of sea salt, and black pepper to taste. Mash the potatoes with a masher or fork. Add the reserved cooking water a tablespoon at a time, as needed, to loosen the mash. Mix in the parsley if using. Serve.

Fennel & Tomato Gratin

Things You Need

5 medium fennel bulbs, stalks removed (see Ann's tips)

1 cup homemade breadcrumbs, or to taste

¾ cup finely grated Parmesan cheese

Black pepper, to taste, Freshly ground

2 tablespoons olive oil

For the Quick Tomato Sauce,

2 tablespoons olive oil

1 1/2 pounds ripe plum tomatoes (about 6-8), coarsely chopped (See Chef Tips)

1 to 2 cloves garlic, smashed and thinly sliced lengthwise

1 small dried red pepper, seeds removed (optional)

1/2 teaspoon salt or to taste

1 tablespoons, freshly grated Parmesan cheese (optional)

Instructions

Preheat the oven to 350 degrees F. Prepare the q uick tomato sauce as outlined here.

Halve the fennel bulbs and parboil in salted water for about 10 minutes or until they are just soft and slightly translucent looking. Drain. Cut into q uarters. If the bulbs are very large, cut each half into 3 pieces. Set aside.

Toss the breadcrumbs and the cheese together in a bowl. Set aside.

Bring the Quick Tomato Sauce to a boil over a medium high flame in a wide sauté pan. Lower the heat to medium and simmer until the sauce has thickened, about 10 to 15 minutes. Set aside.

Spread a thin layer of tomato sauce on the bottom of a shallow gratin dish, about â…" cup. Place the fennel cut sides down on top of the sauce in a tight single layer. Pour the rest of the sauce over them and spread evenly.

Sprinkle the fennel with the breadcrumb mixture until you have a generous crust. Drizzle with the olive oil and bake for 30 minutes covered with foil, then 10 minutes uncovered, or until the breadcrumbs are golden.

Roasted Monkfish With Fennel & Tomatoes

Things You Need

1 whole monkfish tail, about 3 pounds (see Chef Tips)

3 cloves garlic, thinly sliced

2 large fennel bulbs

2 tablespoons olive oil, divided

2 cups cherry tomatoes

¼ cup oil-cured black olives

Sea salt, to taste

Instructions

Heat the oven to 425 degrees. Line a baking sheet or large gratin dish with parchment paper.

Take the monkfish tail and with a small sharp paring knife make small slits into the flesh. Into each slit, place slivers of the garlic until used up. Set aside.

Trim the stalks and feathery leaves from the fennel. Save for another use. Cut the bulb into roughly ¼-inch thick slices. Set aside.

In a large bowl, put 1 tablespoon olive oil. Add the fennel slices and the cherry tomatoes. Gently toss to coat. Place the fennel slices onto the prepared baking sheet spread into a single layer. Put onto a center shelf in the oven. Bake for 15 minutes.

Meanwhile, brush the monkfish with half the remaining oil. Add the rest to a skillet and over medium-high heat, q uickly brown the fish on all sides to seal. It won't get very dark.

Take the fennel out of the oven. Turn the heat down to 375 degrees. Move the fennel to the edges, place the monkfish in the middle, and drizzle any oil from the skillet over it. Add the tomatoes. Sprinkle with salt. Bake for 20 minutes then turn the tomatoes and the fish, basting with the pan juices. Add the olives.

Return to the oven and bake for 10-15 minutes more or until the monkfish is firm and cooked through. Serve in slices with the vegetables spooned over it.

Greek Lemon Soup

Things You Need

7 cups chicken stock

1 cup orzo pasta

3 eggs

1 large lemon, juiced

Salt and ground black pepper

Lemon slices, to garnish

Instructions

In a large pot, bring the stock to a boil. Add the orzo and cook for five minutes. Turn off the heat.

In a medium bowl, beat the eggs until frothy, then add the lemon juice and one tablespoon of cold water. Very slowly stir in a ladleful of the hot chicken stock, then add one or two more. With the heat still off, add the egg mixture to the pot and stir well. (See Chef Tip)

Season with salt and pepper and serve immediately, garnished with lemon slices and fresh herbs.

Bacalao Fish Stew

Things You Need

2 tablespoons extra-virgin olive oil

½ teaspoon salt

1 medium onion, chopped

4 cloves garlic, minced

1 poblano or Anaheim chili pepper, deseeded and chopped

1 (14 ounce) can diced tomatoes

2 tablespoons sliced pimento-stuffed green olives

1 tablespoon capers, rinsed

1 teaspoon dried oregano, or 1 tablespoon fresh oregano, chopped

2 whole branches of cilantro, washed well, plus 1 tablespoon chopped

1 pound white fish fillets, such as haddock, tilapia or cod, skinned and cut into 1½-inch chunks

1 avocado, chopped

1 lime, quartered

Instructions

Heat oil in a large high-sided skillet or Dutch oven over medium high heat. Add the onion, sprinkle with salt and cook for a minute, stirring until the onion starts to soften. Turn the heat down to medium-low and sweat, stirring occasionally, until softened, about 5 to 8 minutes.

Turn the heat up to medium-high and add garlic and poblano pepper. Cook, stirring, for 1 minute. Add the tomatoes. Cook, stirring, for 3 minutes. Add the olives, capers, and oregano. Mix well. Lay the cilantro sprigs on top, cover, and turn the heat down to low. Simmer for 20 minutes. If the mixture seems dry, add up to ½ cup of water, 1 tablespoon at a time. Taste stew for salt. At this point, you can set the stew aside until you are ready to add the fish.

Add the fish chunks and mix them into the stew. Cook until the fish is opaque and just flakes with a fork; it should take no more than

10 minutes. Remove from the heat and let the soup sit for 5 to 10 minutes. This will blend the flavors and finish cooking the fish. Remove the cilantro sprigs. Serve with the chopped cilantro, avocado, and lime wedges on the side. To add heartiness, serve the stew with something to sop up the sauce such as crusty wholegrain bread, or Baked Tortilla Chips.

Grilled Tuna with Mediterranean Herbs

Things You Need

1 Tablespoon Italian parsley, chopped

2 Teaspoons oregano, chopped

1 Teaspoon thyme or rosemary, chopped

1 Scallion, white parts and green, finely chopped

2 Tablespoons olive oil

2 Yellow fin tuna steaks, 1" thick, about 1 lb total weight

Instructions

In a dish just large enough to fit the tuna steaks snugly in one layer, mix together the parsley, oregano, thyme, scallions, and oil.

When well blended, lay the tuna steaks on top, turning to coat them all over with the herb mixture. Cover the dish with plastic wrap and leave to marinate in the refrigerator for about 30 minutes, turning them once.

Heat a stovetop cast iron grill. If a drop of water dropped on it evaporates immediately, it's ready. Add the tuna steaks and sprinkle with a little sea salt. Cook 5 minutes on one side then flip and cook the steaks 3-5 minutes on the other. A shorter cooking time on the second side will give you a rarer steak. Carve the tuna into ¼" slices. Serve immediately.

Mushroom Farrotto

Things You Need

2 ounces dried shiitake mushrooms soaked in 3 cups of boiling water

3 tablespoons extra virgin olive oil, divided

1 onion, diced

1 stalk celery, diced

1 carrot, diced

2 cups farro, rinsed, soaked overnight and drained (see Chef Tips)

1 lemon, juiced and mixed with ⅓ cup water

1 cup water or vegetable stock as needed

2 cloves garlic, thinly sliced

2 shallots, thinly sliced

½ teaspoon dried thyme or 1 large sprig of fresh

1 lb baby bella or portobello mushrooms, cut into ¼ " slices

¼ cup freshly grated Parmesan cheese (optional)

2 tablespoons flat leaf parsley, chopped

Instructions

Soak the dried shiitake mushrooms for 30 minutes while you prep the vegetables. Drain the mushrooms and reserve the soaking water. Strain the soak water through a fine sieve (see Chef Tips). Set aside. Take the soaked mushrooms, discard the woody stems, and roughly chop. Set aside.

Heat 1 tablespoon of the olive oil in a Dutch oven over a medium high flame. When it shimmers, add the onion, celery, and carrot. Sprinkle with salt and cook, stirring until the onion is translucent and the vegetables have softened, about 5 minutes.

Add the drained farro. Cook until the juices in the pan are absorbed. Add the lemon-water mixture and mushroom soaking water, and cook until the farro is "al dente" — tender but still a little chewy — and the water has been absorbed, about 30 minutes. If the farro is dry but still underdone, add the additional water or stock, ¼ cup at a time.

Meanwhile, in a saute pan, heat the remaining olive oil over medium-high heat. Add the garlic, shallots, and thyme. Saute until the shallots start to color, about 3 minutes. Add the chopped dried mushrooms, cook 1-2 minutes, then add the sliced fresh mushrooms. Sprinkle with salt and cook until they wilt, about 5-8 minutes. Cover the pan and turn off the heat. Let the mushrooms steam for 5-10 minutes or until the farro is cooked.

Stir in the sauteed mushroom-mixture and all its juices into the cooked farro. Stir the grated cheese, if using. Taste for salt. Garnish with chopped parsley and serve immediately.

Roast Chicken With Olives, Shallots & Prunes

Things You Need

1 cup whole pitted green olives

½ cup prunes, q uartered

4 medium shallots, quartered

1 large lemon, cut in half, then q uartered

1 teaspoon olive oil

Salt, to taste

2 teaspoons ground cumin

2 teaspoons salt

2 teaspoons paprika

1 teaspoon cayenne pepper

½ teaspoon turmeric

1 tablespoon olive oil

1 (3 pound) whole chicken, q uartered

1 cup water

1 tablespoon red wine vinegar

1 bay leaf

Instructions

Preheat the oven to 350 degrees.

Spread the olives, prunes, shallots, and lemon in the bottom of a deep roasting pan. Drizzle with 1 teaspoon of olive oil and salt.

Mix the cumin, salt, paprika, cayenne, and turmeric together. Rub evenly onto the chicken.

Heat 1 tablespoon of olive oil over medium-high in a wide skillet. Brown the chicken in batches, turning to brown all sides. Place the chicken on top of the olive mixture in the roasting pan. Once all the chicken has been browned, add the 1 cup of water and 1 tablespoon of vinegar to the skillet over high heat. Scrape up the bits at the bottom of the pan and cook until half has evaporated. Pour this into the roasting pan.

Roast for 20 to 30 minutes or until all the chicken is cooked through. Let rest, then serve with Basic Couscous.

Citrus Thyme Roasted Chicken

Things You Need

1 (3½ – 4 pound) whole chicken

1 blood orange, sliced thin

3 tablespoons olive oil

salt and pepper

1 lemon, sliced thin

2 garlic cloves, peeled

8 sprigs of thyme

Instructions

Preheat oven to 400 degrees.

Pat chicken dry and set on a baking dish breast-side up.

Loosen the chicken skin with fingertips. Slide blood orange slices under the chicken skin.

Rub the chicken with olive oil and season with salt and pepper. Season inside the cavity with salt and pepper. Place the lemon slices, thyme and the garlic inside the cavity. Tie the chicken legs together with kitchen twine to close the cavity.

Place the baking dish in the center rack of the oven ,and bake for about an hour or until the temperature of the chicken reaches 165 degrees when poked with a meat thermometer.

Let rest for 10 minutes and serve.

Chickpea Cucumber Toast

Things You Need

1 (15 ounce) can chickpeas, drained and rinsed

1 tablespoon lemon juice

1 ½ teaspoons olive oil

1 tablespoon parsley, chopped

1-2 tablespoons Greek yogurt

Salt and pepper, to taste

6 slices of whole wheat bread

1 English cucumber, sliced

Instructions

In a medium sized bowl, mash chickpeas with a potato masher or fork. Mix in lemon juice, olive oil, and parsley. Season with salt and pepper.

Toast bread slices until golden brown.

Divide the chickpea mixture between the 6 pieces of toast and spread evenly. Top the toast with cucumbers.

Apricot Almond Cake

Things You Need

8 tablespoons butter at room temperature, plus 1 tablespoon butter for pan

⅓ cup fine brown sugar, plus 1 tablespoon for pan

1 (14-ounce) can apricot halves, drained, syrup reserved

2 large eggs, at room temperature

¼ teaspoon orange flower water (optional)

½ cup whole wheat pastry flour (see Chef Tip)

½ cup almond flour

½ teaspoon sea salt

1 teaspoon baking powder

2 tablespoons milk, as needed

2 tablespoons sliced almonds, toasted for garnish

Instructions

Preheat the oven to 375 degrees.

Grease the skillet or cake pan with butter and liberally smear the bottom with the extra tablespoon of butter. Sprinkle with the extra tablespoon of sugar. Arrange the drained apricots in the pan, cut side up, neatly and tightly in a single layer, reserving any leftovers or discarded broken fruits. Set aside while you make the batter.

Put the softened butter, sugar, eggs and orange water, if using, into a large mixing bowl. Sift the whole wheat pastry flour, almond flour, salt and baking powder over it. Beat together with an electric mixer until well blended. If the mixture seems stiff, add a tablespoon of milk or a little of the reserved apricot syrup to bring it to dropping consistency {--|--} where a small amount of the batter will fall off a spoon if gently shaken.

Spoon the batter gently over the apricots with a spatula and smooth to cover them. Bake on a middle shelf for about 30 minutes or until a toothpick comes out clean.

While the cake is baking, take an immersion blender and liq uidize any discarded apricots with the reserved syrup. Add a few drops of orange flower water, if desired. Pour into a small saucepan and gently simmer until the syrup thickens by about a third. Set aside in a jug.

Let the cake sit for 5 minutes. Run a knife round the edges to loosen it, then set a plate over the top and turn the whole thing upside down. Tap all over the bottom of the skillet and lift it off the cake. You will have a cake with caramelized apricot topping sitting on the plate. Sprinkle with toasted almonds. Serve warm with the reserved sauce, and for extra richness, a dollop of marscarpone or Greek yogurt.

Celery Root & Potato Soup

Things You Need

1 pound celery root

1 tablespoon unsalted butter

1 small onion, diced

2 tablespoons Greek yogurt, plus more for garnish

1 pound Idaho potatoes (about 2 large spuds), cut into a ½-inch dice

6 cups low sodium chicken stock

1 tablespoon chopped parsley, for garnish

Salt and pepper, to taste

Instructions

Cut off the gnarly top and the bottom of the celery root. Peel and rinse it well to remove any remaining dirt. Halve and cut each half into a ½ inch dice. Set aside.

Sauté the onion in the butter over a medium high heat until they are soft and have browned slightly.

Add the yogurt and fry until all the liq uid has evaporated. Add a grind or two of black pepper. Fry for a minute or so more.

Add the potatoes and celery root and cook for a couple of minutes, then add the stock. Bring the soup to a boil, lower heat to a simmer, cover and cook until the vegetables are tender. Purée with an immersion blender or in batches in a blender.

Serve garnished with chopped parsley and a dollop yogurt, if desired.

Chicken & Butternut Squash Tagine

Things You Need

2 tablespoons olive oil

2 cups chopped onion

2 garlic cloves, minced

¼ teaspoon salt

2 teaspoons ground cumin

1 teaspoon paprika

1 teaspoon ground turmeric

¼ teaspoon ground cinnamon

¼ teaspoon ground ginger

1 pound skinless, boneless chicken breast, cut into bite-sized pieces

8 ounces (about 2 cups) peeled and cubed butternut squash

⅓ cup halved pitted black oil-cured olives

⅓ cup pitted prunes, chopped

½ cup fresh cilantro leaves and flat-leaf parsley leaves (optional)

Instructions

Heat oil in a Dutch oven or other heavy pot over medium heat. Add onion; sprinkle with salt. Cook, stirring occasionally, until soft and golden, for about 8-10 minutes. Raise the heat to medium high and stir in the garlic. Cook until it becomes fragrant, about 1 minute.

Stir the ground cumin, paprika, turmeric, cinnamon, and ginger into the onions. Cook for 1 minute, stirring constantly. Add the chicken pieces and stir to coat with the spices. Add 1 cup of water. Stir well, scraping off any of the spice mixture stuck to the bottom of the pan into the sauce.

Add sq uash, olives, and prunes; bring to a boil. Cover. Reduce heat to medium-low, and simmer 10-15 minutes or until sq uash is tender and the chicken cooked through. Taste for salt. Garnish with cilantro and parsley. Serve with Basic Couscous.

Chicken & Turkey Meatballs

Things You Need

2 tablespoons olive oil

1 clove garlic, sliced

2 sprigs fresh thyme, leaves stripped from the stems

2 shallots or ½ an onion, finely diced

1 large egg

⅓ teaspoon ground cinnamon (optional)

⅓ teaspoon ground nutmeg (optional)

Salt and pepper

1 cup whole-grain breadcrumbs, plus,

2 tablespoons whole-grain breadcrumbs

2 tablespoons stock or water

¼ pound ground chicken

¼ pound ground turkey

2 tablespoons finely chopped parsley

1 tablespoon ground almonds (optional)

2 cups tomato sauce, heated through

Instructions

Heat 2 teaspoons of the oil in a small skillet over a medium-high flame. When it is hot, add the garlic. Cook until golden, then discard. This will flavor the oil.

Add the thyme to the oil and cook for 1 minute. Add the shallots and turn the heat down to medium-low, and cook until the shallots start to turn golden. Do not let them burn! Set aside.

Beat the egg. Add cinnamon, nutmeg, salt, and pepper and mix well.

In a separate bowl, mix the cup of breadcrumbs with the stock or water.

In a large bowl combine the ground chicken and turkey with the cooked shallots and parsley, mix with a spatula. Mix in the beaten egg. Gradually add in the ground almonds, if using, and then the breadcrumbs, a little at a time. If using ground almonds, you may not need all of the breadcrumbs. Mix well. Add a little water if it seems too stiff or dry.

Lay a sheet of parchment or wax paper on your work surface and sprinkle with 1 tablespoon of breadcrumbs. Using a full tablespoon, spoon the meat mixture it into balls with your hands then gently roll them in the breadcrumbs. Set aside on a plate. Repeat until all the meat mixture is used up.

Coat 2 teaspoons of the olive oil in a skillet over medium-high heat. When the oil is hot cook the meatballs in batches until they are browned all over, drizzling a little more oil into the pan as needed. Set them aside on a clean plate as you cook them. At this point, you can freeze the meatballs for a future meal.

For pasta, when all the meatballs are cooked, tip them into the tomato sauce and cook gently for about 10 minutes. Eat with the whole-grain pasta of your choice and a grating of fresh Parmesan.

Spanish Garlic Soup

Things You Need

2 tablespoons olive oil

¼ pound any stale bread, crusts removed, cut into 1/2 inch cubes (see Chef Tips)

4 garlic cloves, minced

½ teaspoon hot pimentón (smoked paprika)

Salt, to taste

4 cups chicken stock or vegetable stock

4 eggs, poached (see our Poached Eggs

Instructions

In a medium-sized pot, heat the olive oil over medium-high heat. Add the cubed bread and cook for 5 minutes, stirring often, until the bread is lightly browned. Add the garlic, pimentón, and a pinch of salt. Stir well, and cook for 3 minutes.

Pour in the stock, bring to a boil, then reduce heat to a simmer. Cook for 15 minutes, or longer for a sweeter less pungent garlic flavor.

Ladle soup into bowls and serve topped with a freshly poached egg.

Grilled Chicken Breasts in Rosemary Marinade

Things You Need

Marinade:

2 tablespoons extra virgin olive oil

2 medium sprigs rosemary, leaves stripped and roughly chopped

2 cloves garlic, smashed and roughly chopped

1 teaspoon lemon zest

Juice of 1 large lemon

Chicken:

2 skinless, whole chicken breasts, halved (see Chef Tips)

⅓ cup water

Salt, to taste

Instructions

Mix together all the marinade ingredients.

Place the chicken in a baking dish that's large enough to hold all the pieces tightly. Pour the marinade over the chicken, turning it to make sure it is well coated. Cover and leave in the fridge for an hour, longer if you can, turning the pieces from time to time.

Heat the grill or broiler.

Turn the chicken in the marinade one more time to coat it evenly and set it on a plate. Sprinkle with a little sea salt.

Grill the chicken 5-8 minutes a side, depending on the thickness of the breasts. When it's done, the juices should run clear. Let them sit a minute or two before serving.

Put the remaining marinade in a small saucepan. Add ⅓ cup water and a pinch of salt. Bring to a boil and cook down, stirring, until the mixture has reduced by about half.

Slice the breasts crossways and drizzle the sauce over them through a small strainer. Serve!

Pan-Fried Marinated Tofu

Things You Need

For the marinade:

3 tablespoons olive oil

⅔ cup chopped fresh cilantro

¼ cup chopped fresh mint

½ cup lemon juice

6 garlic cloves, minced

1 teaspoon ground cumin

½ teaspoon smoked paprika

¼ teaspoon cayenne (optional)

2 teaspoons agave syrup

1 (1-pound) block extra-firm tofu, cut into ½-inch slices

For cooking and serving:

1 tablespoon olive oil

Cilantro and mint, chopped for garnish

Instructions

Add all marinade Things You Need and sliced tofu to a resealable plastic bag. Marinate tofu for at least 20 minutes or overnight.

Preheat 1 tablespoon of olive oil in a large saucepan over medium-high heat. When oil starts to ripple, add tofu to pan, being careful not to overcrowd the pan, which can steam instead of fry the tofu. If tofu doesn't sizzle immediately when adding to the pan, remove it and wait another minute.

Cook tofu on both sides until golden, about four minutes on each side. Right before removing tofu from pan, pour in extra marinade from the bag and cook down until it's slightly thickened. Transfer cooked tofu to a plate with sauce and garnished with more fresh herbs. Serve immediately with a crisp salad, roasted vegetables, and/or brown rice.

IDEAS FOR DINNER

Mediterranean Chicken Skillet Dinner

Things You Need

1 teaspoon dried oregano, divided

½ teaspoon black pepper, divided

1 pinch Salt to taste

4 (6 ounce) skinless, boneless chicken breast halves

2 tablespoons olive oil, divided

1 small lemon, cut into 8 slices

¼ (8 ounce) jar chopped, drained oil-packed sun-dried tomatoes

2 large garlic cloves, minced

1 (8.8 ounce) pouch UNCLE BEN'S® READY RICE® Roasted Chicken Flavored Rice

⅓ cup unsalted chicken stock

1 (6 ounce) package fresh baby spinach

1 ounce feta cheese, crumbled (Optional)

2 tablespoons toasted pine nuts

Instructions

Combine 1/2 teaspoon oregano and 1/4 teaspoon pepper, adding salt if desired. Sprinkle evenly over top of chicken.

Heat 1 tablespoon oil in a 10-inch skillet over medium-high heat. Add chicken to pan, seasoned-side down. Cover and cook until browned, about 6 minutes. Turn chicken over, and top each breast with 2 lemon slices. Cover and cook 6 minutes or until a thermometer inserted in thickest part of chicken registers 165 degrees F. Place chicken on a plate; cover loosely to keep warm.

Heat remaining 1 tablespoon oil in skillet over medium-high heat. Add sun-dried tomatoes and garlic; cook 1 minute, stirring constantly. Add rice, chicken stock, remaining 1/2 teaspoon oregano, and remaining 1/4 teaspoon pepper to skillet. Gradually add spinach, stirring gently until spinach wilts. Nestle chicken breasts back in skillet. Sprinkle with cheese and pine nuts.

Sheet Pan Vegetable Dinner with Feta

Things You Need

¼ cup olive oil

2 small zucchini, sliced

2 small carrots, chopped

2 red bell peppers - cored, seeded, and cut into chunks

2 potatoes, peeled and cut into 1/2-inch cubes

15 cherry tomatoes

15 black olives

4 green onions, chopped

2 cloves garlic, pressed or minced

2 teaspoons dried oregano, or to taste

2 teaspoons dried thyme, or to taste

salt and freshly ground black pepper to taste

2 sprigs rosemary

2 bay leaves

1 (4 ounce) package feta cheese, crumbled

Instructions

Preheat oven to 400 degrees F (200 degrees C). Grease 2 baking sheets with 2 tablespoons olive oil each.

Distribute zucchini, carrots, red bell peppers, potatoes, cherry tomatoes, black olives, and green onions between the 2 baking sheets. Season with garlic, oregano, thyme, salt, and pepper. Place 1 rosemary sprig and 1 bay leaf on each baking sheet.

Bake in the preheated oven until vegetables are lightly browned and easily pierced with a fork, 25 to 35 minutes. Remove from oven, distribute feta evenly between the 2 baking sheets, and return to oven. Bake until feta is slightly melted, 5 to 10 minutes.

Roasted Cod Nicoise

Things You Need

cooking spray

1 ½ pounds small new red potatoes, cut into 1-inch chunks

2 tablespoons olive oil, divided

¼ teaspoon salt

8 ounces thin French-style green beans, trimmed

1 ½ teaspoons coarse-ground Dijon mustard

⅛ teaspoon salt

⅛ teaspoon ground black pepper

4 (6 ounce) cod fillets

3 tablespoons prepared black olive tapenade

6 lemon wedges, or to taste

1 cup grape tomatoes, halved

2 tablespoons chopped fresh parsley

Instructions

Preheat the oven to 400 degrees F (200 degrees C). Line an extra-large rimmed baking sheet with parchment paper. Coat parchment with cooking spray.

Toss potatoes in a bowl with 1 1/2 tablespoon oil and 1/4 teaspoon salt. Transfer to the prepared baking sheet and roast for 20 minutes.

Toss green beans in bowl with remaining 1/2 tablespoon oil, mustard, remaining 1/8 teaspoon salt, and pepper. Push potatoes to one side of the baking sheet. Lay beans and fish separately on the other side. Spread 3/4 tablespoon tapenade on each fillet.

Bake until cod is no longer translucent and flakes easily with a fork, 12 to 15 minutes. If vegetables need more time, transfer cod to a plate and cover with foil to keep warm. Roast vegetables 5 to 10 minutes more.

Serve with lemon wedges, tomatoes, and parsley.

Vegan Green Bean, Tomato, and Basil Sheet Pan Dinner

Things You Need

2 cups baby potatoes

3 tablespoons olive oil, divided (Optional)

2 cups cherry tomatoes

2 cups 1-inch cut fresh green beans

4 cloves garlic, minced

2 teaspoons dried basil

1 teaspoon flaked sea salt (such as Maldon®)

1 (15 ounce) can garbanzo beans, drained and rinsed

2 teaspoons olive oil, or to taste (Optional)

salt and ground black pepper to taste

Instructions

Preheat the oven to 425 degrees F (220 degrees C). Line a jelly roll pan with aluminum foil.

Toss potatoes with 1 tablespoon olive oil in a medium bowl. Pour into the prepared pan.

Roast in the preheated oven until tender, about 30 minutes.

Toss cherry tomatoes, green beans, garlic, basil, and sea salt with 2 tablespoons olive oil.

Remove potatoes from the oven, push them to one side of the pan, and add the tomato and green bean mixture. Roast until tomatoes start to wilt, 15 to 20 minutes more.

Remove from the oven and pour into a serving dish. Stir in garbanzo beans, add 2 teaspoons olive oil, and season with salt and pepper.

Sheet Pan Salmon and Bell Pepper Dinner

Things You Need

2 tablespoons olive oil

4 (3 ounce) fillets salmon fillets

2 red bell peppers, chopped

1 yellow bell pepper, chopped

1 onion, sliced

Sauce:

6 tablespoons lemon juice

3 tablespoons olive oil

2 tablespoons water

1 tablespoon maple syrup

5 cloves garlic

1 ½ teaspoons salt

1 ½ teaspoons red pepper flakes

1 teaspoon ground cumin

½ bunch fresh parsley, chopped

1 lemon, sliced

Instructions

Preheat oven to 400 degrees F (200 degrees C). Grease a sheet pan with 2 tablespoons olive oil.

Place salmon fillets, red and yellow bell peppers, and onion on the prepared sheet pan.

Combine lemon juice, 3 tablespoons olive oil, water, maple syrup, garlic, salt, red pepper flakes, cumin, and parsley in a small bowl. Drizzle 2/3 of the sauce over the Things You Need on the sheet pan.

Bake in the preheated oven until salmon is cooked through and flakes easily with a fork, 10 to 15 minutes.

Serve with lemon slices and remaining sauce.

Vegetarian Sheet Pan Dinner with Chickpeas and Veggies

Things You Need

2 (15 ounce) cans chickpeas, rinsed and drained

½ butternut sq uash - peeled, seeded, and cut into 1-inch pieces

1 onion, diced

1 sweet potato, peeled and cut into 1-inch cubes

2 large carrots, cut into 1 inch pieces

3 medium russet potatoes, cut into 1-inch pieces

3 tablespoons vegetable oil

1 teaspoon salt

½ teaspoon ground black pepper

1 teaspoon onion powder

1 teaspoon garlic powder

1 teaspoon ground fennel seeds

1 teaspoon dried rubbed sage

2 green onions, chopped (Optional)

Instructions

Preheat the oven to 350 degrees F (175 degrees C). Grease a large sheet pan.

Place chickpeas, butternut sq uash, onion, sweet potato, carrots, and russet potatoes on the prepared sheet pan. Drizzle with vegetable oil and toss to coat.

Combine salt, black pepper, onion powder, garlic powder, ground fennel seeds, and rubbed sage in a bowl. Sprinkle over vegetables on the sheet pan and toss to coat.

Bake in the preheated oven for 25 minutes. Stir and bake until vegetables are soft and lightly browned and chickpeas are slightly crisp, 20 to 25 minutes more. Season with additional salt and black pepper to taste, and top with chopped green onion before serving.

Sheet Pan Mediterranean Frittata

Things You Need

1 (12 ounce) package chicken sausage, sliced in 1/2-inch rounds

1 ½ cups sliced zucchini

1 cup grape tomatoes, halved

½ cup diced red onion

1 tablespoon olive oil

12 large eggs

1 cup milk

¾ teaspoon kosher salt

½ teaspoon ground black pepper

¼ cup crumbled feta cheese

1 tablespoon chopped fresh dill

Instructions

Preheat the oven to 400 degrees F (200 degrees C).

Place sausage, zucchini, grape tomatoes, and red onion on a rimmed baking sheet. Drizzle with olive oil and toss to combine. Spread into a single layer.

Roast in the preheated oven until browned around the edges, about 7 minutes.

Remove sausage mixture from the oven and reduce heat to 375 degrees F (190 degrees C).

Whisk eggs, milk, salt, and pepper together in a bowl. Pour evenly over the sausage mixture and sprinkle feta cheese over top.

Return to the oven and bake until eggs are set, 17 to 20 minutes.

Sprinkle with dill and serve.

Mediterranean Chicken Sheet Pan Dinner

Things You Need

¼ cup extra-virgin olive oil

lemon, juiced

2 tablespoons balsamic vinegar

1 teaspoon dried tarragon

1 teaspoon dried oregano

1 teaspoon paprika

1 teaspoon salt

½ teaspoon black pepper

4 chicken thighs with skin

1 small red onion, sliced into petals

8 mini bell peppers, halved lengthwise and seeded

1 pound baby potatoes, halved

1 lemon, sliced

¼ cup crumbled feta cheese

¼ cup fresh parsley, chopped

8 pitted kalamata olives

Instructions

Preheat the oven to 425 degrees F (220 degrees C). Line a large rimmed baking sheet with aluminum foil.

Whisk olive oil, juice of 1 lemon, vinegar, tarragon, oregano, paprika, salt, and pepper together in a large bowl. Add chicken thighs, onion, baby bell peppers, and potatoes. Stir until everything is evenly coated.

Transfer vegetable-chicken mixture to the prepared baking sheet and spread in an even layer. Scatter lemon slices over the vegetables, making sure to leave the chicken uncovered so that the skin will brown.

Bake in preheated oven for about 40 minutes. Remove from oven and top with feta, parsley, and olives.

Sheet Pan Ratatouille

Things You Need

1 large eggplant, cut into 1/2-inch cubes

2 zucchinis, cut into 1/2-inch slices

2 heirloom tomatoes, cut in wedges

1 white onion, cut into 1/2-inch-thick rounds

1 red bell pepper, cut into 1/2-inch strips

4 cloves garlic

2 tablespoons olive oil

2 tablespoons chopped fresh rosemary

1 teaspoon salt

½ teaspoon ground black pepper

1 tablespoon balsamic vinegar

Instructions

Preheat oven to 400 degrees F (200 degrees C). Line a baking sheet with parchment paper.

Place eggplant, zucchinis, tomatoes, onion, bell pepper, and garlic in a single layer on the prepared baking sheet. Drizzle with olive oil, rosemary, salt, and pepper; toss vegetables until well coated.

Roast in the preheated oven until slightly tender; about 20 minutes. Mix and roast for another 12 minutes. Reduce heat to 300 degrees F (150 degrees C) and cook until vegetables begin to caramelize; about 10 minutes. Drizzle with balsamic vinegar.

Greek Chicken and Potato Bowl

Things You Need

2 pounds boneless, skinless chicken thighs

2 teaspoons kosher salt

2 teaspoons freshly ground black pepper

1 teaspoon dried rosemary

1 teaspoon dried thyme

2 teaspoons dried oregano

¼ teaspoon red pepper flakes

1 pinch cayenne pepper

4 cloves garlic, minced

1 large lemon, juiced

¼ cup olive oil

2 medium russet potatoes, peeled and cut into 1-inch cubes

1 pinch kosher salt

1 splash olive oil

For the Dressing:

¼ cup red wine vinegar

⅓ cup olive oil, or to taste

1 large lemon, juiced

salt and freshly ground black pepper to taste

2 tablespoons chopped flat-leaf (Italian) parsley

2 tablespoons chopped fresh oregano

For the Salad:

2 cups cubed English cucumber

2 cups halved cherry tomatoes

½ cup sliced red onion

1 cup cubed feta cheese

4 cups mixed salad greens

Instructions

Combine chicken thighs, 2 teaspoons kosher salt, pepper, rosemary, thyme, oregano, red pepper flakes, cayenne, garlic, lemon juice, and 1/4 cup olive oil in a large mixing bowl. Toss very thoroughly to combine, making sure the chicken thighs are completely and evenly coated with the marinade.

Wrap in plastic and marinate in the refrigerator for 6 to 12 hours.

Preheat the oven to 475 degrees F (245 degrees C). Line a baking sheet with foil and grease generously with olive oil.

Meanwhile, halve potatoes lengthwise; slice each half into 3 eq ual pieces. Dice into cubes and set aside.

Transfer chicken thighs to the prepared sheet pan smooth-side up, spacing evenly. Reserve any excess marinade in the bowl.

Add the potatoes to the bowl the chicken was in, along with a splash of olive oil and a large pinch of salt. Toss well to coat evenly. Scatter potatoes onto the chicken and distribute as evenly as possible in between the chicken thighs to fill any empty spaces.

Roast in the center of the preheated oven until the chicken is cooked through, about 35 minutes. Remove chicken to a plate or dish and cover. Chicken can be cut into bite-sized pieces if desired.

While chicken and potatoes are cooking, whisk red wine vinegar, olive oil, lemon juice, salt, and pepper together for dressing. Taste and adjust vinegar or oil as needed. Whisk in parsley and oregano.

Toss the potatoes in the chicken fat and pan drippings, and return to the oven until well browned and crusty, 10 to 15 minutes. Let potatoes rest for a few minutes before removing them with a spatula.

To make bowls, toss together cucumbers, tomatoes, red onions, feta cheese, chicken, potatoes, and dressing until evenly combined. Serve on top of a bowl of greens.

Shrimp and Vegetable Sheet Pan Dinner

Things You Need

1 red onion, coarsely chopped

1 red bell pepper, chopped

1 cup sliced fresh mushrooms

1 zucchini, chopped

3 tablespoons olive oil, divided

salt and freshly ground black pepper to taste

¼ teaspoon paprika

1 pound fresh shrimp, peeled and deveined

1 teaspoon lemon zest

½ teaspoon garlic powder

Instructions

Preheat the oven to 425 degrees F (220 degrees C).

Combine red onion, bell pepper, mushrooms, zucchini, 2 tablespoons olive oil, salt, pepper, and paprika on a sheet pan and toss well to combine.

Roast in the preheated oven until vegetables are softened, about 15 minutes.

While vegetables are roasting, combine shrimp, 1 tablespoon olive oil, lemon zest, garlic powder, salt, and pepper in a bowl. Toss to combine.

Remove roasted vegetables from the oven and add shrimp to sheet pan, spreading everything out evenly in one layer. Return to oven and bake until shrimp are pink and cooked through, 5 to 7 minutes.

DELICIOUS SOUPS AND STEWS

Best Ever Split Pea Soup

Things You Need

1 tablespoon olive oil

2 cups chopped onion

2 cups chopped carrot

2 cups finely chopped celery

1 ½ teaspoons minced garlic

1 cup yellow split peas

1 cup green split peas

8 cups fat-free chicken broth

1 ½ teaspoons salt-free seasoning blend (such as Mrs. Dash®)

1 teaspoon salt

Instructions

Heat oil in a Dutch oven over medium heat. Add onion, carrot, celery, and garlic; cook and stir until onion is translucent, 5 to 7 minutes. Stir in broth, split peas, and seasoning blend; cover and bring to a boil. Reduce the heat and simmer, stirring freq uently, until peas are tender, about 2 1/2 hours. Purée with an immersion blender and serve.

Chicken Vegetable Soup

Things You Need

4 cups water

6 bone-in chicken thighs

2 tablespoons olive oil

2 carrots, chopped

½ onion, diced

4 cloves garlic, chopped

1 ½ teaspoons salt

1 (32 ounce) carton chicken broth

1 head broccoli, trimmed and chopped

¼ head cauliflower, trimmed and chopped

1 zucchini, trimmed and chopped (Optional)

Instructions

Place water and chicken thighs in a pot. Bring to a boil; reduce heat and simmer until chicken is tender, about 30 minutes. Occasionally skim off scum as it forms.

Heat olive oil in a large pot over medium heat. Cook and stir carrots and onions until they begin to soften, 3 or 4 minutes. Stir in garlic and salt; cook for 1 minute.

Transfer chicken and cooking water to large pot. Add chicken broth. Bring mixture to a boil; reduce heat to low. Cover, leaving lid slightly ajar, and simmer at least 1 hour or up to 4 hours. Remove from heat.

Transfer chicken to a work surface. Remove skin, bones, and cartilage. Shred chicken meat using 2 forks. Return chicken to pot. Add broccoli, cauliflower, and zucchini. Bring back to a simmer over medium-high heat. Reduce heat so soup gently simmers. Cook until vegetables are tender, 20 to 30 minutes.

Greek Lentil Soup (Fakes)

Things You Need

8 ounces brown lentils

¼ cup olive oil

1 medium onion, minced

1 large carrot, chopped

1 tablespoon minced garlic

1 quart water

2 bay leaves

1 teaspoon dried oregano

1 pinch crushed dried rosemary (Optional)

1 tablespoon tomato paste

salt and ground black pepper to taste

1 teaspoon olive oil, or to taste

1 teaspoon red wine vinegar, or to taste (Optional)

Instructions

Place lentils in a large saucepan; add enough water to cover by 1 inch. Bring water to a boil and cook for 10 minutes; drain.

Heat olive oil in a saucepan over medium heat. Add onion, carrot, and garlic; cook and stir until onion has softened and turned translucent, about 5 minutes. Pour in lentils, then add 1 q uart water, bay leaves, oregano, and rosemary. Bring to a boil. Cover and reduce heat to medium-low; simmer for 10 minutes.

Stir in tomato paste; season with salt and pepper. Cover and simmer, stirring occasionally, until lentils have softened, 30 to

40 minutes. Add additional water if soup becomes too thick. Drizzle with olive oil and red wine vinegar to serve.

Sweet Potato Black Bean Soup

Things You Need

1 (32 fluid ounce) container vegetable broth

4 cups peeled and cubed sweet potatoes

1 (15 ounce) can reduced-sodium black beans, rinsed and drained

1 cup mild picante sauce

1 (12 ounce) jar roasted red peppers, coarsely chopped

¼ cup chopped cilantro

1 tablespoon smoked paprika

2 medium limes, juiced

Instructions

Combine vegetable broth and sweet potatoes in a pot over medium-high heat. Bring to a boil and cook until sweet potatoes are softened, about 7 minutes.

Meanwhile, combine black beans and picante sauce in a blender; blend until smooth.

Add the black bean mixture and roasted red peppers to the soup. Reduce heat. Add cilantro, smoked paprika, and lime juice. Stir soup and cook until heated through, 5 to 7 minutes.

Vegan Creamy Mushroom and Farro Soup

Things You Need

1 tablespoon olive oil

1 small onion, finely diced

2 stalks celery, roughly chopped

3 carrots, roughly chopped

1 teaspoon finely chopped garlic

1 teaspoon dried basil

1 teaspoon dried oregano

1 pound mixed mushrooms, roughly chopped (cremini, portobello, white)

1 teaspoon salt

½ teaspoon freshly ground pepper, or to taste

¼ cup fresh celery leaves, chopped

1 (32 ounce) carton unsalted vegetable stock

¾ cup farro

2 tablespoons tomato paste

2 tablespoons low-sodium soy sauce (such as Bragg®)

1 (14 ounce) can coconut milk (such as Aroy-D)

Instructions

Heat olive oil in a pot over medium heat. Add onion, celery, and carrots. Cook until onion is soft and translucent, 3 to 5 minutes. Add garlic, basil, and oregano and cook for another 30 seconds. Mix in mushrooms, salt, and pepper. Cover and cook, stirring occasionally, over medium-low heat for 10 minutes.

Uncover and add celery leaves, vegetable stock, farro, tomato paste, and soy sauce. Simmer until farro is cooked, 25 to 30 minutes.

Pour in coconut milk and heat until soup is warmed through, 5 to 10 minutes.

Ribollita (Reboiled Italian Cabbage Soup)

Things You Need

2 cups dry cannellini beans

4 cups water

3 (32 ounce) cartons chicken broth

5 cloves garlic, minced

4 sage leaves

2 bay leaves

1 teaspoon salt

½ cup olive oil

2 onions, diced

3 carrots, peeled and sliced

3 large stalks celery, chopped

2 potatoes, peeled and cut into chunks

1 ½ cups cabbage, coarsely chopped

1 bunch Swiss chard, trimmed and chopped

1 bunch kale, trimmed and chopped

1 (14.5 ounce) can diced tomatoes

12 (1/2-inch-thick) slices French bread, lightly toasted

salt and freshly ground black pepper to taste

1 ½ cups grated Parmesan cheese for topping

½ cup olive oil

Instructions

Sort and rinse the beans before placing them in a large pot with the water. Bring to a boil over medium-high heat and cook 5 minutes. Turn off heat, cover, and let stand 1 1/2 hours. Drain.

Place the beans, chicken broth, garlic, sage leaves, bay leaves, and salt in a large pot. Bring to a boil over medium-high heat. Reduce heat to low and simmer until beans are tender, about 2 hours. Cool. Remove 1 cup of beans. Discard the bay leaves and sage leaves. Blend the remaining bean mixture with a hand mixer until smooth. Set aside.

Heat the olive oil in a large pot over medium-high heat. Add the onions; cook and stir until transparent, about 10 minutes. Combine the carrots, celery, potatoes, cabbage, Swiss chard, and kale with the onions. Stir in the tomatoes. Season with salt and pepper to taste. Cover, and cook until greens have wilted, stirring at least once, about 20 minutes. Stir in the pureed bean mixture, and cook 40 minute until the mixture thickens. Stir in the reserved beans. Adjust seasonings to taste. Add the toasted bread slices; cook until bread is soaked, about 10 minutes longer. Cool, and refrigerate overnight.

Reheat the soup over low heat until heated through, about 20 minutes. Serve each serving garnished with 2 tablespoons Parmesan cheese and a drizzle of olive oil.

Spicy Lime Avocado Soup

Things You Need

2 skinless, boneless chicken breasts

1 tablespoon olive oil

1 large white onion, chopped, divided

3 limes, juiced

1 cup chopped cilantro, divided

2 jalapeno peppers, halved and thinly sliced

3 cloves garlic, minced

4 cups water

2 tablespoons reduced-sodium chicken bouillon powder

3 large firm-ripe avocados, cut into chunks

¼ cup crumbled q ueso fresco, or to taste

Instructions

Bring a small pot of water to a boil. Add chicken; boil until an instant-read thermometer inserted into the center reads at least 165 degrees F (74 degrees C), about 7 minutes. Drain.

Run cool water over chicken to speed cooling process. Shred or finely slice chicken.

Heat olive oil in a large pot over medium heat. Add 1/2 onion, lime juice, 1/2 cup cilantro, jalapeno peppers, and garlic until onion is slightly greenish in color, about 5 minutes.

Combine 4 cups water and bouillon powder in a small bowl. Pour into the pot. Let cook until just heated through, about 5 minutes. Stir chicken into the pot.

Ladle soup into 4 bowls. Top with remaining 1/2 onion, 1/2 cup cilantro, avocado, and q ueso fresco.

Sweet Vegan Butternut Squash Soup

Things You Need

3 tablespoons olive oil

1 medium butternut sq uash, halved and seeded

1 medium sweet potato, halved

4 cloves garlic, minced

8 leaves fresh sage, or to taste

1 tablespoon maple syrup

4 cups vegetable broth, divided

2 bay leaves, or more to taste

1 cinnamon stick

1 tablespoon fresh thyme

1 teaspoon salt

ground black pepper to taste

Instructions

Preheat the oven to 400 degrees F (200 degrees C). Coat a baking sheet with olive oil.

Place butternut squash and sweet potato cut-sides down on the baking sheet.

Bake in the preheated oven until easily pierced with a knife, 45 to 50 minutes. Remove from the oven and let sit until cool enough to handle.

While sq uash and potato are cooking, heat 3 tablespoons oil in a skillet over medium-high heat. Add garlic and fresh sage and cook until garlic is browned and sage is crispy, 3 to 5 minutes. Remove sage to a paper-towel lined plate. Transfer garlic to a blender.

Scoop out the flesh of the butternut squash and potato using a spoon and transfer to the blender with garlic. Discard squash and potato skins. Add maple syrup and 1 cup vegetable broth to the blender and process until smooth, 1 to 2 minutes.

Strain through a sieve to remove any lumps and transfer into a large pot. Add remaining 3 cups vegetable broth, bay leaves, cinnamon stick, 1 tablespoon thyme, and salt. Bring to a simmer over medium heat, then reduce heat to low and simmer for 30 minutes. Season with pepper and sprinkle with crushed sage leaves.

Creamy Italian White Bean Soup

Things You Need

1 tablespoon vegetable oil

1 onion, chopped

1 stalk celery, chopped

1 clove garlic, minced

2 (16 ounce) cans white kidney beans, rinsed and drained

1 (14 ounce) can chicken broth

¼ teaspoon ground black pepper

⅛ teaspoon dried thyme

2 cups water

1 bunch fresh spinach, rinsed and thinly sliced

1 tablespoon lemon juice

Instructions

In a large saucepan, heat oil. Cook onion and celery in oil for 5 to 8 minutes, or until tender. Add garlic, and cook for 30 seconds, continually stirring.

Mediterranean Fish Soup

Things You Need

2 (14 ounce) cans chicken broth

1 (14.5 ounce) can diced tomatoes, drained

1 onion, chopped

½ green bell pepper, chopped

1 (8 ounce) can tomato sauce

½ cup orange juice

½ cup dry white wine

2 ½ ounces canned mushrooms

¼ cup sliced black olives

2 bay leaves

2 cloves garlic, minced

1 teaspoon dried basil

¼ teaspoon fennel seed, crushed

⅛ teaspoon ground black pepper

1 pound medium shrimp - peeled and deveined

1 pound cod fillets, cubed

Instructions

Place broth, tomatoes, onion, bell pepper, tomato sauce, orange juice, wine, mushrooms, olives, bay leaves, garlic, basil, fennel seed, and black pepper into a slow cooker. Cook on Low until vegetables are crisp-tender, 4 to 4 1/2 hours.

Stir in shrimp and cod. Continue cooking until shrimp are opaque, 15 to 30 minutes. Discard bay leaves before serving.

SECTION 9: IN SUMMARY!

Psoriasis, a persistent autoimmune ailment, presents as patches of skin that manifest with distinctive characteristics such as reddish spots and persistent itching. These patches may emerge in localized areas or spread across the entire body, yet it's vital to emphasize that psoriasis is not communicable. While the precise etiology of psoriasis remains elusive, it is believed to arise from a complex interplay of environmental factors, genetic predispositions, and a compromised immune system.

Categorized into five distinct types—plaque, guttate, inverse, erythrodermic, and pustular—psoriasis primarily manifests as plaque psoriasis, affecting a significant majority of individuals with the condition. This subtype is typified by the formation of red patches covered with silvery-white scales, commonly observed on the forearms, scalp, shins, and navel. Genetic susceptibility compounded by environmental triggers contributes to the onset of psoriasis, as evidenced by studies indicating a higher concordance rate among identical twins compared to non-identical twins.

Psoriasis symptoms often exacerbate during colder months, and despite ongoing research efforts, a definitive cure remains elusive. However, various treatment modalities exist to manage symptoms effectively. Triggers such as stress, smoking, excessive alcohol consumption, skin infections, streptococcal throat infections, and certain medications—including those prescribed for bipolar disorder and hypertension—can exacerbate psoriasis or incite its onset.

The impact of psoriasis extends beyond physical symptoms, significantly affecting patients' emotional well-being and social interactions. Individuals grappling with psoriasis often experience diminished self-esteem, depression, and may withdraw from social engagements. Seeking medical consultation upon experiencing symptoms is crucial, as early diagnosis and intervention can mitigate the condition's progression.

Ongoing research underscores the role of a compromised immune system, particularly the aberrant activation of T cells targeting healthy tissue, in precipitating psoriasis. Additionally, a familial predisposition to the condition heightens the likelihood of its development, particularly among individuals with a parental history of psoriasis. Moreover, individuals with pre-existing viral or bacterial infections, such as HIV, face an increased susceptibility to psoriasis.

Lifestyle factors such as stress, alcohol consumption, and obesity are recognized as exacerbating elements in psoriasis. Anything that influences the delicate balance of the human immune system can potentially serve as a risk factor for the development or exacerbation of psoriasis.

Central to managing psoriasis is arresting abnormal cell proliferation, a cornerstone of treatment strategies. While specific symptoms may vary among individuals, common manifestations include dry, cracked skin prone to bleeding, persistent itching, joint swelling, and the presence of silvery scales atop red skin patches. Given the chronic and fluctuating nature of psoriasis symptoms, consistent medical monitoring and personalized treatment plans are essential for optimal disease management and improved quality of life.